# FIBROMYALGIA RELIEF

## Successful Self-Care Strategies And Effective Natural Remedies

Joseph K. Egbebike, PhD.,PT

FIBROMYALGIA RELIEF

Copyright © 2016 by Joseph K. Egbebike, PhD.,PT

Southstar Publishing Company, 5549 Ft Caroline Rd, #110, Jacksonville, FL. 32277

# Medical Disclaimer

The information and treatment protocols in this book are based upon the research, personal and clinical experience of the author. This book is not intended to be a substitute for medical care and advice. You are advised to consult a physician or healthcare provider in matters relating to your health, including those which require diagnosis and medical attention.

In particular, you are advised to consult a qualified medical practitioner if you are taking any medication or plan to stop taking any particular medication. Because of possible withdrawal reactions, you are advised to find a sympathetic qualified physician to assist you.

The publisher does not advocate the use of any particular healthcare protocol, but believes that the information contained in this book should be made available to the public. The publisher and the author are not responsible for any adverse reactions due to the use of any suggestions or remedies discussed in this book

# Table of Contents

# Expanded Table Of Contents

The impact of methylation on human life • Glutathione and antioxidation • Homocysteine: the SAM e adversary • Are there other substances that can promote the methylation process?

Chapter 10 How Does SAM-e Relieve Fibromyalgia Syndrome?

A theoretical model for the probable action of SAM e in the relief of fibromyalgia symptoms • Probable FMS causative factors in which SAM e may be able to mediate • Factors and symptoms for which SAM e brings relief • SAM e and gene expression abnormality • SAM-e and sleep disorders • SAM e, abnormal brain function and neurotransmitter regulation • SAM e and autoimmune disorders • SAM e and depressive moods and fatigue • SAM e, muscle pain and tender points • SAM e and migraine headaches • Recent scientific studies on the effects of SAM e on fibromyalgia

Chapter 11 Other Uses of SAM e

SAM e and osteoarthritis • SAM e and the liver • SAM e and brain diseases like Parkinson's and Alzheimer's • SAM e and cardiovascular disease

Chapter 12 How to Take SAM e for Fibromyalgia

Buying the right SAM e • Toxicity • Dosage • Possible side effects • Contra-indications • Optimal dosage recommendation • Dosage for fibromyalgia with depressive moods • Dosage for other conditions

Chapter 13 Ideas About How to Safely Come Off Your Addictive Medications. What to Do About Withdrawal Symptoms

# INTRODUCTION

Surprisingly, there are still some nice things that can be said about pain. We are able to feel pain because we are alive. We learn how to live fully because we have survived pain and suffering.

No one has been able to escape suffering. It will continue to be part of our human heritage. Pain, in one form or another, will find and embrace us. It has taught us much more about ourselves and others than anything else.

Through pain and suffering we learn to appreciate life and what we have, and we develop more empathy for those who suffer. So pain now and then is normal. Those who can't feel it, like in diabetes, are in danger of injury to their body parts. But constant unrelenting pain is another matter. Christine, for example, can't remember a day without pain. It feels to her like she has a perpetual flu.

Christine's problems started about 8 years ago when she suffered a whiplash neck injury in a motor-vehicle accident. A drunken motorist had slammed his car into the back of her car as she waited at a stop sign. Since then, the symptoms have multiplied and seemed to take on lives of their own.

Even though she is 38, she now feels like 60. She has been forced to quit her job as a schoolteacher. She and her husband of 9 years barely survived on what he made from his construction business. This financial problem has not helped her condition. She has recently been denied disability benefits by the Social Security Administration, the reason being that her pain and symptoms were not sufficient enough and lacked proof of any disability that would preclude a regular employment. The SSA suggested some possible vocational and job alternatives.

Before her accident, Christine had had a very active lifestyle. Even though she was diagnosed with some form of scoliosis as a child, she had pushed herself through several athletic activities since 7th grade. She kind of felt that if she pushed herself hard enough, the scoliosis would go away. And in fact it did. It did not progress.

But then the generalized body pain started. Outwardly, she looked fine, but she felt terrible. Besides the pain, there was constant fatigue, unrefreshing sleep. Cold weather made her symptoms worse.

Christine had run the gamut of doctors and therapists, taken countless MRIs, CAT scans, x-rays and blood work. No one seemed to understand what was happening to her. Then she visited a rheumatologist, who diagnosed her condition as fibromyalgia.

According to the doctor, the whiplash neck injury was the precipitating factor for all these symptoms. Of the 13 so-called "tender points" tested, Christine had about 11 really painful spots. The doctor prescribed a daily does of 25 mg of amitriptyline, to be taken together at night with 400 mg of ibuprofen.

This would help her sleep better. This treatment helped, but she had needed to increase the dosages. Gradually, Christine noticed that she had developed other problems like diarrhea, dizziness and vomiting.

She had also gained more weight and gotten more depressed. When she tried to decrease the dosage or even come off it totally, her problems became worse and she had to quickly get back on her previous dosage. Christine felt powerless, almost imprisoned in her body.

She lost interest in everything. Avoided socializing. She knew no one could possibly understand what she was going through. Her relationship with Andy, her husband, was suffering also and they became more distant. She simply lost all interest in any intimacies.

Christine's story is fictional, but it serves to illustrate a malady that is common to over 6 million Americans, mostly women. We know from several scientific studies that fibromyalgia is not a psychiatric disorder or just "in the head" of these sufferers.

Rather, any depression is usually as a result of frustration at a very elusive and debilitating sickness. We now know that it is a chronic condition characterized by generalized pain, tender points and a host of other symptoms.

It can also come with a retinue of other problems like chronic fatigue syndrome, arthritis, lupus, etc. Presently, there is no single FDA-approved drug that can cure it. Doctors are not even sure what causes it or how it progresses. Treatment therapies are mostly empirical. With no dosage guidelines, doctors rely on a trial-and-error method, using drugs that are effective for similar conditions.

But fibromyalgia is unique, because there are no "real" symptoms that can show up as evidence in lab tests. So patients become frustrated and depressed. Tranquilizers and antidepressants are prescribed at random. These in time add on their own adverse side effects.

But antidepressants and all the other drugs may not be the "fix-all" that they are purported to be. According to the internationally noted psychiatrist Dr. Breggin, the human brain is much more complex than the universe. Modern medicine has not even begun to unravel the mysteries of the brain – its intricate internal structure, interconnections, the exact nature of the numerous chemical messengers known as neurotransmitters.

According to Dr. Breggin in his book *Your Drug May Be Your Problem*, "[T]he knowledge that we have about the effects of psychiatric drugs on the brain is largely limited to test-tube studies of biochemical reactions utilizing ground-up pieces of animal brain. We simply do not understand the overall impact of drugs on the brain."

According to an April 1998 *Journal of the American Medical Association* report, medications, even when taken as intended, have the potential of serious side effects that can cause disability or may even be fatal.

Most importantly they can take away the independence and spontaneity of life, and the will to engage the sufferer's inner healing resources. For a chronic condition like fibromyalgia with no known cure, with a multitude of symptoms, I think that an adequate treatment approach should include a multi-faceted approach that aims at empowering the sufferer with natural and self-help strategies.

It is presumptuous for any clinician to make a 15-minute decision about medications that will drastically alter a patient's life. The so-called studies on which the efficacy of these medications are based may just be marketing efforts of powerful, profit-crazy drug companies.

It is therefore with great excitement that I learned about SAM-e (pronounced Sammy). Since then, I have read all I could on the subject. The more I read, the more amazed I became about the general ignorance in this country about this supplement.

SAM-e, as we have learned, has been used for decades by doctors in Europe with excellent results. Evidence from several scientific studies suggest that SAM-e can be a good substitute for the tricyclic antidepressants currently used to treat fibromyalgia.

In one study reported in the *Scandinavian Journal of Rheumatology*, 800 mg of SAM-e taken daily for 6 weeks improves "disease activity" in fibromyalgia patients. It relieves pain, morning stiffness and depressive moods. This is in agreement with several others studies on fibromyalgia and related conditions. SAM-e was shown by these studies to work as well as and even faster than conventional antidepressants. Most importantly, it does so without the usual adverse side effects of those antidepressants.

Recently, the field of alternative or integrative medicine has gained prominence. A recent study in the *Journal of the American Medical Association* reported that Americans spend about $27 billion yearly on alternative medicines, herbs and books.

According to Jack Daniel of the Center for Traditional Acupuncture in Columbia, Maryland, "People don't look for alternatives if they're satisfied with what they've got." People are not so happy with the status quo. They realize there is much more to their lives beyond physical symptoms.

They realize that conventional medicine is an impressive science. The information superhighway explosion called the "Internet" now lies at their disposal, a lot of information about alternative self-help strategies that they were not privy to before. And luckily medicine, whose turf is being invaded, has been keeping pace with these developments, although reluctantly.

Of course, there is a lot of hype out there. This is expected in a free-for-all unregulated turf that has the promise of quick profits. But we have certainly come a long way from the days of Dr. John Cohausen. Did you know he prescribed the "breaths of little girls" as an anti-aging elixir? According to David Louis in his book *2201 Fascinating Facts*, Dr. Dohausen actually wrote the following prescription: take one pound of gum olibani, two ounces of styrae, myrrh and several other herbs, mix, burn and inhale while at the same time imbibing the exhalations of the nearest little girl.

On a serious note though, I sincerely think that SAM-e, combined with perhaps very low doses of regular medications, lots of exercise, relaxation techniques, proper nutrition, better stress management and other self-help strategies is the way to go for fibromyalgia.

I have tried to arrange the chapters of this book in a logical sequence. My main aim in writing this book is to empower you, the fibromyalgia victim, with enough information on the subject to wrest your life back from fibromyalgia and chemical dependency.

After reading this book, it is my hope you would have learned the following lessons:

- Basic facts about SAM-e and fibromyalgia, so you can discuss intelligently with your doctor about trying out SAM-e
- Side effects and withdrawal symptoms of your current medications
- How to safely come off your addictive medications
- Correct dosage and type of SAM-e to take
- Several self-help strategies to better manage your stress, muscle soreness, chronic fatigue, sleep and other problems
- Appropriate nutritional supplements for fibromyalgia
- An illustrated fibromyalgia-specific fitness and exercise guide

- How to successfully apply for disability benefits if you need to

# Chapter 1: Understanding Fibromyalgia Syndrome (FMS)

The constant complaint of fibromyalgia sufferers is that everywhere and everything hurts – the weather, cold water or the cold draft that rushes in through the open window. In Christine's case, the pain starts from the neck and radiates down to the arms and the back. Each morning, instead of feeling refreshed like everyone else, rather, she feels tired.

In Debbie's case, it was a headache that didn't seem to respond to anything. It gets frustrating when it seems your physician and relatives don't seem to understand what you are going through. You sometimes have the feeling that they may all be thinking you are malingering. Other fibromyalgia sufferers have described symptoms similar to what feels like a perpetual flu and muscle soreness.

## SO WHAT IS THIS THING CALLED FIBROMYALGIA?

Prior to the 1990 American College of Rheumatology definition, there had been some controversy about what it really was. Some had called it "fibrositis," which of course meant an inflammatory process in the fibrous connective tissues.

But soon the term was considered a misnomer, since muscle biopsy reports do not indicate an inflammatory process. Eventually, a consensus was reached by the American College of Rheumatology to call it "fibromyalgia." The word "syndrome" was added to denote its multi-symptomatic nature.

According to the College's criteria, fibromyalgia syndrome (FMS) was defined as a chronic disorder characterized by persistent and widespread muscle soreness, stiffness, chronic fatigue and many other symptoms, especially well-defined painful spots called "tender points."

Other problems of FMS include problems with concentration or memory difficulty called "fibro-fog." X-rays, CAT scans and blood analysis do not show abnormalities. Most often, sufferers are asked to take things easy, do more exercise and generally try not to mind it. As time goes on and the complaints continue, family support may waver.

The spouse gets more irritable as the condition forces lifestyle changes. Soon some fibromyalgia sufferers develop depressive moods, as the problem seems to take over their lives. They become less active and sociable, hoping to resume their lives as soon as things get better. But it doesn't get better and they drift more and more into depression and inactivity with all the attendant problems.

Then the physician starts experimenting with anti-anxiety drugs and antidepressants and these people become addicted. The side effects of the drugs add additional problems. If the fibromyalgia sufferer attempts to discontinue medications, they are hit with additional problems known as "withdrawal symptoms." Patients often move from one doctor or therapist to another – each with a different idea that doesn't seem to work. These sufferers often feel trapped inside their bodies, with no freedom in sight.

### Who Gets Fibromyalgia?

About 80% of those who suffer from fibromyalgia are women between ages 25 and 55. No one really knows why it affects mostly women. According to Dr. Goldenberg, a professor of medicine and chief of rheumatology, about 3 to 6 million Americans are affected. In fact, it is regarded as the most common cause of generalized muscle soreness which affects about 2% of the general population. Men, when affected, don't get it as hard as women.

According to available statistics, fibromyalgia affects people between the ages of 20 and 60 years with a peak at about age 35.

Children and Fibromyalgia

A so-called "juvenile primary fibromyalgia" is reported in about 2% of school children, mostly girls. Symptoms in children include irritability and attention deficit in school. Others complain of allergy problems and painful joints.

## Economic Cost of Fibromyalgia

Dr. Wolfe and associates determined from their studies that it costs the nation about $16 million in missed work and disability payments or poor work performance.

## Can Fibromyalgia Be Inherited?

A CBS Health Watch article reports that about 28% of siblings of fibromyalgia sufferers (mothers) also developed symptoms. Another study claims 66% of parents of children with fibromyalgia exhibited some sore muscular pain. But most researchers agree that studies could not conclusively determine whether psychological conditioning by regular contact played any role or whether it is in fact due to genetic factors.

## Who Is At Risk?

Anybody really, but mostly women between the ages of 25 and 55, especially those with a medical history of trauma. Christine's whiplash neck injury had been her fibromyalgia triggering factor. Other factors might include constant mental aggravation due to frequent relationship discords, or physical, emotional and sexual abuse. Those with low stress tolerance or poor coping capacity are particularly susceptible to fibromyalgia.

## How Does Fibromyalgia Progress?

We deduce from several long-term studies that fibromyalgia is chronic in nature, often alternating from "good days" to "bad days." Some have been forced to stop walking altogether.

Although fibromyalgia is chronic, it does not appear to be progressive or fatal. Many people have been known to improve following a well-controlled self-help remedies, stress management and fitness programs. Children with fibromyalgia usually improve faster than adults, probably due to their resilient spirit and active lifestyle.

# Chapter 2: Common Symptoms And Associated Conditions

There are many diseases that can be confused with fibromyalgia. These have similar symptoms but are technically not fibromyalgia. This distinction will become more explicit hen we discuss the American College of Rheumatology's diagnostic criteria later on in this text.

Similar conditions that are easily confused with fibromyalgia syndrome include:

- Chronic fatigue syndrome
- Lyme disease
- Lupus
- Polymyalgia rheumatica
- Rheumatoid diseases
- Sjögren's syndrome

We shall now briefly describe these conditions, their similarities with fibromyalgia and how you can tell them apart. Please note that your fibromyalgia can also come with a whole retinue of diseases and you may in fact have fibromyalgia syndrome with arthritis or Sjögren's syndrome, etc.

And we think this is often the case in most instances. People with autoimmune problems or connective tissue diseases like polymyalgia, etc. are particularly prone to fibromyalgia. Often many physicians fail to check for these other conditions and as a result patients may not improve or respond to medications as they should.

### Chronic Fatigue Syndrome

Many of the symptoms of chronic fatigue syndrome (CFS) are quite similar to those of fibromyalgia syndrome (FMS). A major difference is that while fatigue is the dominant symptom in CFS, widespread pain and tender points are more predominant in FMS. A similarity, though, is that both FMS and CFS occur in similar age groups of 20 to 50, and mostly in women. According to Dr. Carol Jessop, both conditions may have similar symptoms like:

- chronic fatigue
- memory problems
- depressive moods
- frequent urination
- cold extremities
- sleep abnormality
- problems with balance
- muscle spasm
- dry mouth
- headaches
- muscle aches

Another difference is that cognitive impairment is more pronounced in CFS than in FMS.

In general, chronic fatigue syndrome is characterized by extreme and continuous fatigue. A little physical exertion usually provokes a fatigue that can incapacitate patients for days. There is no clinical testing for CFS. Instead physicians endeavor to exclude other conditions before making a diagnosis of chronic fatigue syndrome.

Lyme Disease

Lyme disease is caused by a bacteria called Borrelia burydorferi, usually transmitted by tiny deer ticks. It got its name from the Lyme community in Connecticut, where it was first discovered and named in 1975.

Symptoms begin as a large red spot on the thigh or buttocks, trunk or armpit and expands to about 6 inches in diameter. Other smaller red spots may appear later. Other symptoms include fatigue, chills and fever, muscle and joint pain, headaches or neck stiffness.

Diagnosis of Lyme disease can be difficult as the bacteria is difficult to culture. So diagnosis is usually based on a history of exposure to tick infestation and a measuring of the level of antibodies to Borrelia in the blood of patients.

**Lupus**

Lupus, which affects about 2 of every 1000 persons, may be mistakenly diagnosed with fibromyalgia. Common symptoms of this disease include joint pains, fatigue, muscle soreness and skin rashes. It has been shown in research studies that about 30% of lupus patients also have fibromyalgia.

Differences with fibromyalgia include: evidence of true joint swelling (arthritis), mouth sores, fever, skin rashes, hair loss, and organ disease like blood in urine. Other characteristics of lupus include elevated blood sedimentation rates, depressed white blood cell count, and increased anti-DNA antibodies.

Fibromyalgia, on the other hand, does not have any of the above findings and is characterized by more widespread pain, tender points and possibly irritable bowel syndrome.

### Polymyalgia Rheumatica (PMR)

One difference is that PMR occurs in people over age 50, and like fibromyalgia is more common in women than in men. PMR is a condition that is characterized by severe pain and stiffness in the neck and in the muscles of the shoulders and hips. It can be accompanied by another condition called temporal (giant cell) arteritis. Other symptoms of PMR include fever, weight loss and depression. Onset of symptoms can be either sudden or gradual. A blood test usually reveals a high erythrocyte sedimentation rate.

### Rheumatoid Diseases

Rheumatoid arthritis is an autoimmune condition characterized by symmetrical inflammation of joints, usually of the hands and feet, and the eventual disruption of interior joint structures like cartilage, bones and ligaments.

A major difference with fibromyalgia is that in fibromyalgia there is neither a joint inflammation nor disruption.

Sjögren's Syndrome

Many patients have been diagnosed with both Sjögren's syndrome and fibromyalgia syndrome. Sjögren's syndrome's cause is unknown. It is characterized by a distinctive type of dry mouth and dry eyes. There are tooth problems, oral infections, difficulty in swallowing. It is an autoimmune problem, prevalent in middle-aged women. Additionally, Sjögren's disease may be associated with arthritis, muscle inflammation, and thyroid and kidney problems. Sometimes there is fatigue and sleep disorder.

A diagnostic criteria for Sjögren's disease is evidence of keratoconjunctivitis sica (abnormality and deficiency of tear ducts) and autoimmune problems. There is increased sensitivity to light. Corneal erosion can develop with prolonged dryness of the eyes.

Common Symptoms of Fibromyalgia and Associated Disorders

The following are some common problems fibromyalgia sufferers may have, with their approximate incidence in percentages. Please note that several investigators report different percentages of incidence. (You should take these numbers only as rough estimates.)

- Widespread muscle pain or soreness (100%)
- Fatigue (85%)
- Morning stiffness (75%)
- Headaches (70%)
- Depression and anxiety (20%–50%)
- Irritable bowel syndrome (IBS) and other
- Abdominal and digestive problems (70%)
- Restless legs syndrome (RLS) (31%)
- Cognitive and memory impairment problems (71%)
- Irritable bladder syndrome (12%)
- Pelvic pain (40%)
- Temporomandibular joint dysfunction (TMJ) (25%)

- Vision problems (95%)
- Hearing problems (31%)
- Respiratory problems (33%)
- Hypersensitivity to so-called environmental stressors (50%)
- Raynaud's phenomenon (38%)

Widespread Muscle Pain and Soreness

There may be many other reasons why fibromyalgia sufferers "hurt all over, all the time," but the commonest reasons are:

- Lack of refreshing sleep
- Constant muscle tension

The problem of sleep will be discussed later in greater detail, but in general and under normal situations, the normal muscle micro-trauma is repaired naturally during the deep phase of sleep. Due to absence of this phase in fibromyalgia patients, muscle trauma is not repaired, and this results in the feeling of soreness FMS patients complain about.

Normal muscle tension is the state of readiness of a muscle fiber just before it twitches and performs an action. Due to stress, muscle fibers of muscles of FMS sufferers are constantly twitching – that is, they are always in constant states of readiness, which in the long term places them in permanent states of tension.

Consequently more blood flow, with its oxygen and nutrients, is required to maintain this habitual tension. Unfortunately, this tension constricts the blood vessels, further diminishing the needed blood flow. There is a consequent lack of oxygen and accumulation of harmful by-products of muscle activity called metabolites – like lactic acid. These also contribute to the sensation of pain in the muscles.

**Fatigue**

The cause of fatigue in fibromyalgia and its nature is complex and multifaceted. It is easily triggered off by slight physical exertion, and mental and psychological stress. Scientific evidence indicates fatigue in fibromyalgia is often caused by the following: non-restful sleep; depression and anxiety; lack of physical activity and deconditioning; poor stress management; and hormonal imbalance.

**Sleep Disorders**

There are five (5) phases of sleep in a normal sleep pattern, known as stages 1 to 4 and REM (rapid eye movement). The normal sleep cycle progresses from stage 1 through REM stage, then starts all over again from stage 1 (see figure 2). [note: no figure 1 before this--Patty] Fifty percent of sleep time is spent in stage 2; about 20% in REM stage and the remaining 30% distributed to the other stages. Infants spend most of their time in the REM stage.

**Characteristics of the Stages**

Stage 1: Sleep is light and one can be awakened easily. There are slowed-down eye movements and muscle activity.

Stage 2: Eye movements stop altogether. Brain activity diminish to occasional spikes known as sleep spindles.

Stage 3: Extremely slowed-down brain activity called delta waves interspersed with smaller and faster waves.

Stage 4:    Mostly delta wave activity. Difficult to awaken someone in this phase. This is the deepest sleep phase, which starts in stage 3.

**REM:** This stage is characterized with rapid breathing, which is also shallow and irregular; temporary limb muscle paralysis, rapid eye movements; heart rate increases; there is regular dreaming during this stage.

The initial REM stage occurs after about 70 to 90 minutes of falling asleep. The whole sleep cycle is 90 to 110 minutes. First cycle has a relatively short REM stage and a longer deep sleep phase. As sleep progresses, the REM stage increases while deep sleep stages shorten.

With fibromyalgia patients, there is a sleep disorder called alpha-EEG anomaly. In this problem, the patient falls asleep normally, but the deep phase, ie, stage 4, is often interrupted by awake-like brain activity bursts.

Other sleep disorders include sleep myoclonus (nighttime involuntary jerking of limbs), restless legs syndrome and bruxism (teeth grinding).

Sleep is most restful during the delta or stage 4 phase. It is also called the restorative stage because it is at this stage that "repairing" growth hormones are released from the pituitary gland. This hormone has direct effect on the regeneration of muscle tissue. This is probably why FMS patients feel a muscle soreness and fatigue in the morning.

Morning Stiffness

The FMS patient feels each morning as if her muscles are glued down and immobile. This often persists for more than 30 minutes. The etiology, as I have already explained, is due to lack of restorative sleep among sufferers.

Headaches

Most FMS sufferers complain of migraines. This is defined as a one-sided and throbbing head pain accompanied by nausea and hypersensitivity to light and sound. The headaches are often triggered off by certain kinds of food or strong smells, and may occur during menstruation.

The other type of headache often complained about is called tension headache. It is characterized by pain around the head (hatband) and neck regions. The pain is constant, often precipitated by stress and muscle tension, and usually occurs later in the day.

Recent research studies implicate a high level of substance P as the culprit in headaches of fibromyalgia. As we already know, this substance has some relevance in the etiology of fibromyalgia and may be why fibromyalgia is usually accompanied by headaches and migraines.

Depression and Anxiety

Most researchers believe fibromyalgia is not a psychiatric disorder. Rather, it is a reaction or frustration with fibromyalgia and the lifestyle changes it forces on the sufferers.

Irritable Bowel Syndrome (IBS)

The National Digestive Diseases Department defines IBS as a disorder of the intestines which leads to crampy pain, boating, gassiness, and bowel habit changes. Cause is unknown, and complete cure is yet to be found.

The colon is about 6 feet long and connects the small intestines with the rectum and anus. Its major function is to absorb water and salts from digestive material that enters from the small intestine. Food may remain for several days in the intestine until most of the fluids and salt are absorbed into the body, then the digestive material residue passes through the colon by a pattern of colon movements which further pushes down the material until it can be evacuated as feces. Colon motility is controlled by nerve and hormonal activity.

In irritable bowel syndrome, there is a disorder of the motility of the entire gastrointestinal system and this produces abdominal pain, constipation or diarrhea.

This disorder affects more women than men in a ratio of 3 to 1. It is especially sensitive to stress, diet, certain drugs, hormones and other intestinal irritants.

Normal gut contractions occur at about 6 cycles per minute. In IBS, it is about 3 cycles per minute. Symptoms include difficulty in passing stools, leading to painful diarrhea or constipation, which can also occur interchangeably.

Some foods like chocolate and milk can provoke symptoms. IBS can be more pronounced during menstruation, and perhaps this is why some researchers believe reproductive hormones may be a causative factor.

Restless Legs Syndrome (RLS)

This refers to a problem FMS patients may experience, usually in the evening before bedtime. Sufferers experience uncomfortable sensations like numbness, itching, tingling or crawling in the limbs, sometimes with spontaneous, uncontrollable leg movements.

Cognitive or Memory Impairments (Fibro-fog)

FMS patients often forget things more frequently than normal. There is also decreased attention span and lack of concentration, and they often require more time to process information. The causes of this problem may be attributable to the mental stress and other psychological problems these patients are going through.

Irritable Bladder Syndrome

There is increased urination frequency; a feeling of pain and pressure in the lower abdomen. There may be painful urination and some incontinence.

Pelvic Pain

FMS patients often complain about painful menstruation and frequent pain and discomfort in the pelvic area.

Temporomandibular Joint Dysfunction (TMJ)

FMS patients often experience substantial pain in the face and head, occurring in the area of the temporomandibular joint. This is usually caused by spasms of surrounding muscles and ligaments. There may not be an internal joint problem. This condition is also called myofascial pain syndrome. Pain originates in the ear region and spreads to the rest of the face.

Vision and Hearing Problems

Symptoms include sensations of blurring, bouncing or double vision. Hearing problems may comprise hypersensitivity to certain sounds.

Respiratory Problems

Patients often complain about shortness of breath even when at rest. Breathing pattern can become erratic and irregular with minimal exertion.

Hypersensitivity to So-Called Environmental Stressors

The fibromyalgia patient's senses are highly sensitized and susceptible to several environmental stimuli. Cold water or a cold draft from an open window is known to trigger off a barrage of symptoms.

Known physical stressors include repetitive activities; abnormal postures; prolonged periods in one posture; or sustained isometric position in daily activities like typing or data entry.

FMS patients are known to have poor stress coping ability. They often break up over little problems. They are often described by family members as "cranky" or "nagging."

Raynaud's Phenomenon

This is also called "cold-induced vasospasm." In lay terms, the small blood vessels constrict, thereby decreasing blood flow to the extremities. The fingers turn very white when exposed to cold temperatures.

# Chapter 3: How Is Fibromyalgia Syndrome Diagnosed?

Diagnosing fibromyalgia syndrome may be similar to peeling off the different layers f an onion bulb. Part of the reason why the word "syndrome" is add to it is that it usually comes ith several symptoms and associated conditions.

In order to make a correct diagnosis of fibromyalgia, the rheumatologist or physician must exclude other fibromyalgia-like diseases like lupus, chronic fatigue syndrome, rheumatic diseases, Lyme disease, polymyalgia rheumtica, and Sjögren's syndrome, among others.

Fibromyalgia is unique in that there is no active inflammation like in rheumatic diseases and most tests will usually have negative results. The physician will usually order a whole range of tests to exclude other diseases. Some of these tests include extensive blood work, thyroid and liver function tests, antibody detection tests, sedimentation rates and psychological tests.

Past medical, personal and social histories are conducted to determine issues like past diseases and treatment, physical injuries, episodes of infection, instances of sexual, physical and emotional abuses, nature of current relationships, medical history, etc.

According to the American College of Rheumatology's 1990 criteria, a diagnosis of fibromyalgia syndrome can be made if the following conditions are present:

1.      Widespread or generalized muscle pain in more than one extremity which lsts for more than 3 months.

2.       A minimum of 11 out of 18 tender points. To determine the presence of a tender point, pain must be provoked by a palpation pressure of about 4 km/cm3. Pain must be enough to cause the patient to flinch or pull back. (See figure 3 for anatomic locations of tender points.)

A trigger point can be differentiated from a tender point because a trigger point pain is dull and usually refers to pain in an area that is distal to the area being palpated. Myofascial pain is a localized area of several trigger points.

See the the illustration in the next page.

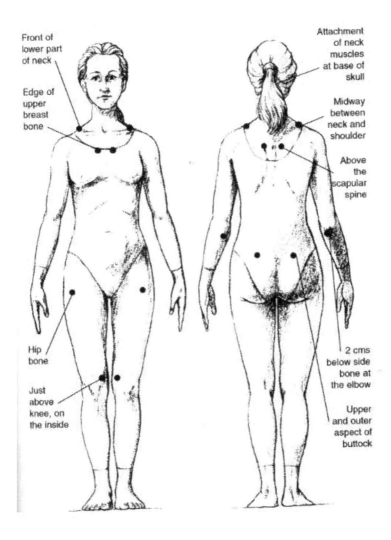

Front of
lower part
of neck

Edge of
upper
breast
bone

Hip
bone

Just
above
knee, on
the inside

Attachment
of neck
muscles
at base of
skull

Midway
between
neck and
shoulder

Above
the
scapular
spine

2 cms
below side
bone at
the elbow

Upper
and outer
aspect of
buttock

# Chapter 4: What Causes Fibromyalgia Syndrome?

Nobody really knows. To date, there is no consensus among fibromyalgia researchers as to a single cause for this syndrome. Rather, there are several theories to explain the causes of a multi-symptom and multi-faceted heath problem. Some of the more important theories include:

- Hereditary factors
- Chronic sleep disorder
- Abnormal brain function and neurotransmitter regulation
- Autoimmune disorder
- Post-traumatic stress disorder
- Trauma like whiplash injury
- Muscle cell abnormality
- Low levels of Vitamin B12
- High homocysteine levels in the cerebrospinal fluid
- Viral infection

Hereditary Factors

A familial predisposition to fibromyalgia has been observed by some investigators. One study reported that 28% of children of mothers with fibromyalgia later developed symptoms of FMS. About 60% developed some kind of fibromyalgia-like muscle pain. Researchers are not so sure about the veracity of this theory. There is some doubt as to whether it is genetic or simply a psychological sensitization due to close association and sympathy with the patient with fibromyalgia.

Chronic Sleep Disorder

Chronic sleep disturbance may be the precipitating cause of fibromyalgia. As we stated earlier, lack of restorative sleep prevents the action of pituitary glands responsible for repairing injured muscle tissue. This leads to muscle hypoxia (oxygen deficiency), and accumulation of metabolites like lactic acid. This problem consequently leads to constant feelings of muscle soreness and pain.

Abnormal Brain Function and Neurotransmitter Regulation

• Brain tissue studies and scans have revealed limited blood flow to pain regulation areas of the brain.

• There may be possible abnormalities with the internal brain system which controls functions like sleep, growth, stress response and depressive moods. These organs include pituitary, adrenal glands and hypothalamus.

• Very high levels of somatomedin C responsible for informing the brain about pain-producing stimuli. High levels of somatomedin C produces increased sensitivity to noxious stimuli in fibromyalgia patients.

• Low levels of the neurotransmitter serotonin and its building material called tryptophan. Neurotransmitters act as chemical messengers between brain neurons. Low levels of these chemical messengers are known to be associated with depressive moods, headaches and migraines, and gastrointestinal problems.

• Elevated levels of substance P in the cerebrospinal fluid have been implicated in fibromyalgia. Animal studies indicate that high levels of substance P lead to what is called "central sensitiza-tion." Substance P is known to decrease the threshold of synaptic sensitivity so that the central nervous system reaction to minor stimuli becomes exaggerated. This is why fibromyalgia patients experience pain very easily.

Autoimmune Disorder

This is a situation when the defective immune system pro-duces agents known as autoantibodies. These autoantibodies at-tack the body's own proteins, mistaking them for harmful foreign proteins. Several of these autoantibodies have been discovered in FMS patients.

Post-traumatic Stress Disorder

Medical and social histories of many fibromyalgia suffer-ers indicate incidents of past sexual, physical or emotional abuse. These incidents create varied anxiety disorders that lead to a full-blown condition known as post-traumatic stress disorder. This condition is characterized by several fibromyalgia symptoms like sleeplessness, mood problems, cognitive problems and muscle pain.

Trauma

Fibromyalgia is often precipitated by trauma. A report in the fibromyalgia newsletter indicates that some scientists in Israel were able to connect the incidence of neck injuries with fibrom-yalgia. In general most fibromyalgia patients usually report a his-tory of past trauma. How trauma provokes fibromyalgia syndrome is not yet fully understood.

Muscle Cell Abnormality

One theory believes that FMS patients have lower levels of ATP (adenosine triphosphate) and phosphocreatine in their muscle cells. These enzymes are responsible for the in-and-out movement of calcium through muscle cells. Calcium motion is a very important process in normal muscle contraction.

With lowered ATP levels, calcium ions are not moved back into the cell after muscle contraction. As a result these fibers remain "frozen" in contraction. They fail to "relax." Some researchers believe the problem may not be within the muscle, but may be a problem within the hormonal and nervous system.

Low Levels of Vitamin B12 and High Levels of Homocysteine in Cerebrospinal Fluid

A Swedish research study, reported in the Scandinavian Journal of Rheumatology, studied 12 female patients with both fibromyalgia and chronic fatigue syndrome. Dr. Regland and associates compared this group to the control group of 18 healthy women. They found that the fibromyalgia and chronic fatigue subjects' cerebrospinal fluid contained a significant amount of homocysteine and a lower amount of Vitamin B12 than that of normal subjects. High levels of homocysteine have been implicated in cardiovascular problems and other diseases. Homocysteine is degraded in enzyme reactions called transsulfuration and remethylation to form methionine, which is the building block for SAM e formation. Vitamin B12 is very important in these enzymatic processes.

Viral Infection

There is a theory that fibromyalgia may be caused by a viral infection. According to Dr. Leon Charton, latent viruses may be reactivated by release of chemicals known as cytokines. This triggers off the "flu-like" symptoms often associated with fibrom-yalgia. Researchers are yet to discover the elusive virus involved in fibromyalgia.

# Chapter 5: Conventional Pharmacological Treatment Of Fibromyalgia

To date, no single medication has been approved by the FDA for the treatment of fibromyalgia symptoms. Because of this, doctors use medications used to treat rheumatic diseases that share some similar symptoms with fibromyalgia.

But unlike rheumatic diseases, fibromyalgia is unique to not having an active inflammatory process. This leads to some difficulty for the physician and risks for the patient, since appropriate dosage guidelines and side effect information are not available to the physician.

According to Dr. Jon Russell, medications are chosen and prescribed based mainly on a pragmatic basis and no particular medication is regarded as a cure.

Sleep Disorders

Common medications used include

- Tricyclics (Elavil, Sinequan, Trazodone, etc.)
- Sedatives and anxiolytics (Xanax, Ambien, etc.)
- Klonopin (prescribed for restless legs syndrome or myoclonus)

Fatigue

- SSRIs (selective serotonin reuptake inhibitors) like Prozac, Zoloft, Paxil, etc. are often prescribed for fatigue and depressive moods

Irritable Bowel Syndrome (IBS)

- Bentyl
- Levsin (used to relieve pain from intestinal spasms, cramps and diarrhea)
- dietary fiber
- Urised (used as a mild anesthetic that affects the nerves that control the action of smooth muscles)

Headaches

- For recurring tension-type headaches, doctors often prescribe a mixture of muscle relaxants and painkillers, or a combination of analgesic-barbiturate and caffeine.
- For persistent migraine, the following are often used: zolmitriptan (Zomig), sumatriptan (Imitrex) and rizatriptan (Maxalt).
- NSAIDs (non-steroidal anti-inflammatory drugs) like Relafen, naproxen, ibuprofen, etc.

According to Dr. Russell, fibromyalgia patients are usually given a combination of NSAIDs and an anxiolygic or a low dose of a tricyclic antidepressant like amitriptyline or cyclobenzaprine.

To avoid the stomach problems caused by NSAIDs, another similar-acting drug called celecoxib (Celebrex) can be used. Celebrex is new in the market, and is being hailed as a "super aspirin." It is as effective as ibuprofen and other NSAIDs.

Mode of Action of Common Drugs Used to Treat Fibromyalgia

Tricyclic Antidepressants

As the name depicts, tricyclics have a 3-ring chemical structure. They were first introduced into the American market in 1960 to be used to relieve depressive moods. Tricyclics work by preventing the reuptake of the neurotransmitters serotonin and norepinephrine, while activating them.

Tricyclics usually require 10 to 14 days on a regular dose to start working. Full effect may be delayed for up to six (6) weeks.

Common tricyclic antidepressants:

- Amitriptyline (Elavil)
- Imipramine (Imavate, Presamine, Tofranil)
- Doxepin (Adapin, Sinequan)
- Desipramine (Norpramin, Pertofrane)
- Protriptyline (Surmontil)
- Clomipramine (Anafranil)

SSRIs (Selective Serotonin Reuptake Inhibitors)

This group of antidepressants have similar effects to tricyclics, except they act to prevent the reuptake of only serotonin. Introduced into the USA markets in 1998, they are used to treat fatigue in fibromyalgia.

Common SSRIs are:

- Fluoxetine (Prozac)
- Sertraline (Zoloft)
- Paroxetine (Paxil)

NSAIDs (Non-Steroidal Anti-Inflammatory Drugs)

NSAIDs have a dual function. First, they affect the prostaglandin system, which is involved in the sensation of pain. Second, they act to reduce inflammation. They are frequently used to reduce fibromyalgia headaches.

Common examples include:

- Relafen
- Naproxen
- Ibuprofen

Anxiolytics – Also Called Sedatives and Tranquilizers

Mostly prescribed to relieve and manage anxiety disorders, they act by relaxing muscles and reducing tension. Used in fibromyalgia to relieve sleeplessness. A common example includes a group called benzodiazepines. Examples of long-acting ones include:

- Diazepam (Valium)
- Alprazolam (Xanax)
- Chlordiazepoxide) (Librium)

Short-acting benzodiazepines include:

- Lorazapam (Ativan)
- Temazepam (Restoril)
- Oxazepam (Serax)

# Chapter 6: Your Medications May Be Doing You More Harm Than Good

According to a recent article in the American Journal of Hospital Pharmacy, the major reasons medications are prescribed include:

- Attempt at enhancing the patient's current quality of life by reducing disease symptoms
- To arrest and regress the disease
- To prevent it from occurring or recurring

But your medication can become a double-edged sword that can cut both ways. It can remove symptoms, and perhaps temporarily mask them, or it can become a foreign agent in the body, having displaced natural ones from their receptor sites, and could even form a totally new adverse compound, further complicating your current problems.

Various medical studies have recently highlighted the issue, which they call "the silent epidemic." According to J. Lazarou and associates' 1998 study reported in the Journal of the American

Medical Association, medications are known to cause serious adverse effects that can cause disabilities or even fatalities. According to the report, 106,000 fatalities occur from drug adverse effects yearly. As a cause f death, it could rank as the fifth highest cause of death. Furthermore, medication-related adverse reactions cost the nation about $85 billion annually.

There is ample scientific evidence that the use of large doses of psychoactive medication for long periods of time for a chronic, vaguely-known condition like fibromyalgia is not good medical practice, especially when alternative patient-empowering remedies can be prescribed.

According to the internationally-known psychiatrist Dr. Breggin, modern medicine does not yet have all the clues about the way the human brain functions. We are yet to understand the nature of its myriad of internal interconnections, the numerous types of chemical messengers known as neurotransmitters.

Most importantly, we don't fully understand how a foreign chemical like an antidepressant can act on so delicate and sensitive a structure as the human brain. According to Dr. Breggin, our knowledge of these issues "is largely limited to test-tube studies of biochemical reactions utilizing ground-up pieces of animal brain.

We simply do not understand the overall impact of drugs on the brain." Some of the so-called studies on which we base our decision to prescribe may very well be marketing propaganda orchestrated by the profit-crazy and influential drug manufacturing companies, who have much at stake in the level of usage.

According to Doctors Gillian Buttler and Tony Hope in their book Managing Your Mind, long-term use of tranquilizers can create the following problems:

1.      It can prevent you from finding long-lasting solutions to your problems. In the short run, they can help you relax, sleep better for the night, cope for a couple of days until the pressure builds up again. However, it does not address the underlying sources of your stress and problems. The medication may just be temporary utopia from the real problems of life that need to be dealt with, such as poor relationship issues, poor stress and muscle tension coping problems.

2.      You end up depending psychologically on your medications. You can't leave home without them. If you realize you did, you will go into a panic, afraid you won't be able to cope without them.

3.      You can get addicted physiologically to your medications. It is usually easier to start than to quit. If you ever try to quit after a long-term usage, you will be hit with a barrage of withdrawal symptoms. Your life is no longer under your control and you get caught up in a vicious cycle you have no hope of escaping.

4.      Long-term antidepressant usage dulls your feelings. People soon notice you are no longer your old self. That natural zest for life, the spontaneous reactions to the vicissitudes of life soon become things of the past.

Too many physicians make rather too quick decisions to prescribe psychoactive drugs. They spend about 15 minutes to make a decision that would change their patients' lives forever. There have been reported instances where physicians changed their prescribing stance or philosophy totally after becoming patients themselves and trying these drugs. How would anybody really know, if they haven't tried them themselves?

The problem, I tend to believe, is aided by the patient's eagerness for a "quick fix" to her problems, as many people are intolerant of the slightest discomfort or pain. And it wouldn't make good business sense for the private-practice physician to resist the patient's craving for tranquilizers.

According to Gabriele Rico in Pain and Possibility: Writing Your Way Through Personal Crisis, "The awareness that pain and possibility are interdependent . . . seeing them as extremes of a single continuum instead of opposites, we begin to see the potential for growth inherent in pain."

Perhaps your pain may be an opportunity for a serious lifestyle conversion in all of its spiritual, emotional and physical ramifications.

# Chapter 7: Adverse Effects And Withdrawal Symptoms AssociatedWith Drugs Used To Treat Fibromyalgia Syndrome

The adverse side effects of all antidepressants can be grouped under the following headings:

- Anticholinergic effects
- Cardiovascular effects
- Renal effects
- Sexual problems
- Otolaryngeal problems
- Skin and allergic reactions
- Central nervous system effects

Anticholinergic Effects

- Memory impairments and sometimes confusion
- Lowered blood pressure
- Episodes of dry mouth
- Bowel problems leading to constipation
- Urination difficulties, like pain or delayed urination
- Blurring of vision and drying of eyes

Cardiovascular Effects

- Low blood pressure resulting in dizziness
- Heart palpitations
- Death can result from cardiac arrhythmias

Gastrointestinal Effects

- Altered bowel movements leading to constipation

- Nausea and vomiting
- Diarrhea
- Patient may gain weight due to increase in appetite and food intake (tricyclics) or lose weight (SSRIs)

Renal Effects

This would include urinary retention and difficulty.

Sexual Effects

- Decreased libido
- Impotence and diminished sexual arousal
- Swelling of the testicles
- Possible enlargement of breasts in both sexes

Otolaryngeal Problems

- Nasal congestion
- Drying of eyes and vision problems
- Glaucoma

Skin and Allergic Reactions

- There may be increased or decreased swelling
- Allergic reactions may occur with skin rashes

Central Nervous System Effects

- Drowsiness
- Impaired ability to concentrate or remember things
- Muscle tremors, slurring of speech, seizures, nightmares and restlessness

Many research studies seem to agree that even though these antidepressants may offer short-term benefits for fibromyalgia sufferers, in the long term they create other serious problems. Even the good short-term benefits wear off within a few months. Some patients like Jean (reported in fibromyalgia news-letter), who has had fibromyalgia for more than 10 years, experienced flashbacks, depressive moods and panic attacks with even a low dose of tricyclics, and she also gained weight. Fibromyalgia sufferers seem to experience fewer side effects with the SSRIs (Prozac, Zoloft) than with the tricyclics (Elavil, Endep, Sinequan, etc.).

In his book Talking Back to Prozac: What Doctors Aren't Telling You About Today's Most Controversial Drug,       [need author]       stated that Prozac can have extreme side effects like "akathisia," restless legs syndrome and the continual needs to pace. Scientific studies confirm this problem in about 10% to 25% of all those on Zoloft.


The restless legs problem may be something fibromyalgia patients should discuss with their doctors if they are on Prozac. Prozac in extreme cases has been linked to suicidal acts and aggressive behaviors towards other people.

Adverse Effects of NSAIDs (Non-Steroidal Anti-Inflammatory Drugs)

Chances for adverse effects increase when two or more NSAIDs are taken together over  a long period of time, or if you take them with alcoholic beverages.

These drugs can cause confusion, dizziness and light-headedness in some people. Others may become extra-sensitive to sunlight, resulting in sunburns with slight exposure.

Serious side effects include gastrointestinal problems – upset stomach, ulcers, stomach cramps, nausea, heartburn or vomiting of blood.

Adverse Effects of Anxiolytics or Tranquilizers Like Benzo-diazepines (Oxazepam, Alprazolam, etc.)

These include:

•        Low blood pressure, dizziness and light-headed-ness

•        Bronchospasm

•        Raynaud's phenomenon – cold fingers and toes

•        Dry mouth and nasal congestion

•        Urination problems

•        Central nervous system effects resulting in disori-entation and confusion; memory problems; frequent episodes of uncontrollable anger

Common Withdrawal Reactions of Antidepressants and An-xiolytics Used to Treat Fibromyalgia Patients

One of the most important reasons not to get on any ad-dictive medication is the withdrawal reactions you will definitely have if you decide to stop. It's like someone deciding to climb a treacherous mountain, who should also consider how she would come down.

There will be no helicopters to carry her off the summit. It is something only she must do. Also be aware that some physicians are not fully informed about withdrawal reactions, coming from a treatment philosophy background of regular prescription and maintenance. According to Mosher and Biroti in their book Com-munity Mental Health:

Principles and Practice, "a sizeable minority of physicians de-nied being confidently aware of he existence of antidepressant withdrawal symptoms." In the final analysis, it is your body, mind and life and you must take charge of them.

All antidepressants and anti-anxiety medications are addictive. It means that you will have what is called "withdrawal reactions" if you try to stop. Your physician may mistakenly interpret this to mean that "you really need this medication and you have to be on it for the rest of your life." This is not always true. And many conscientious psychiatrists will agree with me.

But the withdrawal reactions can be quite significant, depending on what type of medication, dosage and length of time used. The higher the dosage and the longer the time of usage, the more severe the withdrawal reactions will be. These range from emotional to physical reactions, and can be felt within days of stopping the medication.

The short-acting tranquilizers like Ambien, Halcyon or Xanax will cause withdrawal reactions quickly, even in-between doses. Withdrawal reactions usually have opposite effects than those produced by that particular drug. Some of these effects, especially the emotional ones, may last a very long time after completely stopping the medication.

It is possible to stop your addictive medication. You just have to want to stop, and find a psychiatrist who will help you stop by a systematic drug withdrawal program.

Benzodiazepine Withdrawal Reactions (Oxazepam, Xanax, etc.)

These can produce withdrawal reactions even after a few weeks of use. Stopping the use of Xanax, for example, can cause increased anxiety and panic after about 8 weeks of use. In general, depending on dosage and length of time used, benzodiazepams will cause the following withdrawal reactions:

- Flu-like symptoms, chills, shivering
- Stomach upsets like nausea, vomiting and diarrhea
- Sweating
- Fatigue and muscle soreness
- Dizziness
- Blurred vision
- Weight loss
- Psychosis
- Seizures

These reactions may appear in any combination and severity.

Tricyclic Antidepressants Withdrawal Reactions

According to Dr. R.M. Wolfe in his 1997 research study, an attempt to come off tricyclic antidepressants usually triggers off a barrage of "bewildering symptoms." Some of these include:

- Emotional problems like depressive moods, manic episodes, reckless and dangerous behaviors, incidents of very poor judgment, etc.
- Flu-like symptoms
- Gastrointestinal problems like stomach cramps, vomiting and diarrhea, nausea, loss of appetite, etc.
- Memory and other cognitive problems like disorientation

- Uncontrollable muscle movements: spasms, restless legs syndrome
- Sleep problems: insomnia and vivid dreams
- Cardiac arrhythmias that can lead to death if sufficiently severe

SSRIs (Like Zoloft, Prozac, Celexa or Paxil)

Their withdrawal reactions are similar to those of tricyclics with the following additional problems:

- Balance
- Sensory disorders
- Aggressive and impulsive behaviors

Drs. Breggin and Cohen in their definitive book on the subject gave the following case studies.

- A 32-year-old man discontinued Prozac after 6 months of usage and ended up with withdrawal reactions that included painful extensor muscle spasms and uncontrollable tongue-protruding movements.
- A 34-year-old woman tried to stop taking Luvox after she became pregnant. Her withdrawal symptoms included feelings of aggression, like wanting to kill someone.
- Another woman started having problems after reducing her dosage of Zoloft from 100 mg to 50 mg per day. A few days after she started having profound fatigue and depressive moods, and even entertained suicidal thoughts.

# Chapter 8: What Is SAM-e?

SAM e (pronounced as Sammy) is not another new drug product or a herb or hormone, rather it is a naturally occurring substance found evenly distributed in human tissues. SAM e has been in the news lately because it is a harmless supplement which scientists have found to be very beneficial in the treatment of several health conditions including fibromyalgia. The wonder of SAM e is that it works faster and even better than regular drugs without leaving any side effects as drugs do.

Its full biochemical name is "S-adenosyl-L-methionine." Quite a mouthful! To make the pronunciation a little easier, scientists abbreviated it to "SAM e" or SAM." Its biochemical uniqueness can be found in its chemical structure, which is very versatile and allows it to participate in our bodies' several beneficial metabolic processes.

SAM e was discovered and described by Dr. G.L. Cantoni in 1953 at the National Institutes of Health in Bethesda, Maryland. It is formed by the action of ATP (adenosyn triphosphate) and L-methionine or just "methionine," through the enzymatic action of methionine-adenosyl-transferase. Methionine, the building block of SAM e, is an essential amino acid that is usually supplemented by a well-balanced and regular diet of soybeans, seeds and lentils, eggs, and protein-rich foods such as fish and meat, a necessary condition for maintaining other supplements such as the B vita-mins – B12, B6, folic acid and a nutrient called TMG (trimethyl-glycine).

Children have about seven times higher blood levels of SAM e as adults. And men have a higher level than women. The level of SAM e is known to deplete with the aging process and has been implicated as a causative factor in disease states like depression, Alzheimer's and Parkinson's diseases.

As I mentioned earlier on, the versatile chemical structure of SAM e enables it to participate in several of the body's metabolic processes. After ATP, SAM e is the most dynamic single substance in the body. The author of Methyl Magic, Dr. Craig Cooney, goes as far as to claim that without SAM e and the process of methylation which it mediates, there would be no life as we know it.

Methylation is a metabolic process in which SAM e donates its methyl group – a very reactive by-product which is enzymatically transferred to a methyl group acceptor, while leaving behind a by-product called S-adenosyl homocysteine or SAH. This molecule is further degraded by a transfer of its sulfur substrate to other molecules to form several sulfur-containing compounds like cysteine. Cysteine, of course, is the building block for another important substance – an antioxidant called glutathoine, which I shall discuss later.

Even though SAM e was discovered in 1953, it took a while before a stable form of SAM e that can exist outside the body could be produced. In 1973, a guy by the name of A. Fiechi discovered a chemical process that can stabilize SAM e enough so it can be used in clinical trials. Later in 1975, Dr. G. Stramentinoli published the first scientific paper about SAM e's many pharmacological merits. Then in 1976 and 1977, the United States Agencies granted manufacturers patents to produce the stabilized salt forms of SAM e.

Part of the reason SAM e is only recently known in US markets is that most of the scientific investigations and clinical trials were conducted in Europe, notably Italy. This is a part of the world, unlike the USA, that has always been open to alternative forms of healthcare. Nutritionals and supplements have always been parts of the mainstream health care delivery system.

An important milestone in the life history of SAM e in the United States is the passage of an important legislation in 1994 by the Congress. It is called the Dietary Supplement Health and Education Act (DSHEA).

This new law allows drug manufacturers to produce and market any supplement with a good safety record without FDA prior authorization, as long as these companies do not make any outrageous claims about the efficacies of these supplements, which includes SAM e.

They can only hint at its probable benefits. The resultant problem of this law is that there is no longer any quality check scrutiny by the FDA, thereby permitting dishonest producers to flood the markets with substandard products.

The two forms of pharmaceutical grade SAM e currently available are the tosylate (the type commonly imported by US companies) and the butanedisulfonate forms. Because SAM e is absorbed mainly through the intestine, it is usually manufactured in an "enteric coated" tablet form. This allows it to pass intact through the stomach's digestive environment.

SAM e is very unstable, so you must make sure you are buying a well-packaged product, that must be stored properly, usually in a "cool and dry" environment.

# Chapter 9: How Does SAMe Work?

Now that we know what SAM e is and what it is not, the next question is: How does it work its purported magic? The answer lies in the well-known metabolic process called "methylation." According to a well-known methylation scientist, Dr. Craig Cooney, without "methylation," life as we know it will not exist. And another researcher puts it this way: "SAM e is the single most dynamic substance in the body besides ATP."

Methylation is the metabolic process in which SAM e donates one or more of its methyl groups (a carbon atom joined to three hydrogen atoms) to several "acceptor" molecules, thereby producing several beneficial body compounds. One of the most profound impacts of methylation is in the expression or re-activation of DNA, without which of course we would not exist. DNA (deoxyribonucleic acid) is the policeman of our body's zillion cells.

It makes sure each is doing what it is supposed to do. It makes sure genes that can produce cancerous states are kept under lock and key. This is definitely the basic reason why I consider SAM e a very important player in the relief of fibromyalgia syndrome – a condition that most scientists believe is caused and maintained by a central nervous system that has gone berserk.

According to Dr. Cooney, SAM e, through methylation, is involved in the following beneficial metabolic processes among others:

- SAM e mediates in the formation of the body's "biological clock" regulator known as melatonin.

- Assists in the manufacture of adrenaline of the "fight or flight" response fame. When we are faced with danger, adrenaline automatically prepares our bodies for action – the heart beats faster, pumping more blood and oxygen into muscle tissues in readiness for their usage to fight or to run away from danger.

- It assists in the manufacture of several neurotransmitters, like the transformation of L-dopa into dopamine, which is a principal mood regulator.

- SAM e through transmethylation (a term used interchangeably with methylation, being one and the same process), many other substances are created, like L-carnitine, responsible for the transportation of long-chain fatty acids to muscles where they are utilized as fuel.

- Via methylation, creatine phosphate is produced. A supplement form of this is used by athletes who need quick bursts of energy during high-impact sports.

- SAM e through methylation is responsible for removing histamine from our system. Histamine, as we know, is responsible for causing or promoting several allergies and inflammatory reactions.

Scientists believe the full impact of transmethylation is not yet fully understood. Animal studies indicate that the transport of specific nutrients in both bacteria and body cells' membrane vesicles is controlled by the level of methylation.

The story does not end with methylation. After losing its methyl groups, the residue is a compound called S-adenosyl-L-homocysteine (SAH). This compound later loses its sulfur sub-strate to another molecule, with Vitamin B6 as a co-factor to form L-cysteine and several other sulfur-containing compounds. This process is called transsulfuration. Eventually cysteine, through other enzymatic processes, forms the body's major free-radical scavenger, glutathione.

Glutathione

This powerful antioxidant cannot be produced in our body without SAM e's help. In the absence of antioxidants, free radicals will take control and toxins will overwhelm our bodies. A free radical is an excited "bad guy" of our bodies. These molecules are highly charged since they have an odd number of electrons, which forces them to pair up with anything.

They come from harmful products like food preservatives. These free radicals destroy the body through a process known as oxidation. An antioxidant, therefore, is a substance which "ob-structs, restrains or neutralizes" an oxidative product.

Glutathione, together with SAM e, has the highest con-centration in the liver, where glutathione is the greatest detoxifier in the body. The liver is responsible for the elimination of harmful toxins. Low levels of glutathione could lead to liver toxin overload and failure. SAM e therefore has been known to have beneficial effects in the treatment of liver diseases, since it helps produce glutathione.

The Problem of Homocysteine

High levels of homocysteine can lead to another condition called homocystinuria. High homocysteine levels in the blood have been known to cause heart disease. SAM e and homocysteine act from the opposite ends of a precarious balance. A high level of homocysteine is a certain indication of low blood SAM e levels. Therefore, SAM e acts promptly to regulate homocysteine levels.

Are There Other Substances that Can Promote the Methylation Process?

Yes. Trimethylglycine is another methyl group donor. Its limitation, though, is that it is not known to be involved with methylation within brain cells.

As already mentioned, the methylation process declines with the aging process. Low levels of SAM e in the blood invariably lead to higher levels of homocysteine and oxidation. So as we age and SAM e levels in the blood deplete, we will need to supplement with SAM e.

# Chapter 10: How Does SAMe Relief Fi-bromyalgia Symptoms?

Before discussing the several scientific studies that conclusively offer proofs of the beneficial and symptom-relieving effects of SAM e on fibromyalgia, I would like to outline some basic facts that may help explain the puzzle. Fibromyalgia is not a simple condition; rather, it is called a syndrome because there are several other problems associated with it.

One thing seems to be common, though: a kind of faulty amplification of pain and symptoms. This situation would point to a problem that reaches far deep into the basis of life itself – that is, DNA, RNA, polyamines and protein synthesis problems.

As mentioned in earlier chapters, SAM e, because of its great ability to donate a very reactive methyl group, has become the most versatile and dynamic substance in the body besides ATP. Without methylation and transsulfuration, of which SAM e is the main precursor, life would not exist.

So if you are looking for a multifaceted curative agent, SAM e is your answer. It repairs and it replenishes.

A. Probable FMS causative factors in which SAM e may be able to mediate

- Gene expression abnormality
- Sleep disorder

- Abnormal brain function and neurotransmitter regulation
- High homocysteine levels in CSF
- Autoimmune disorder

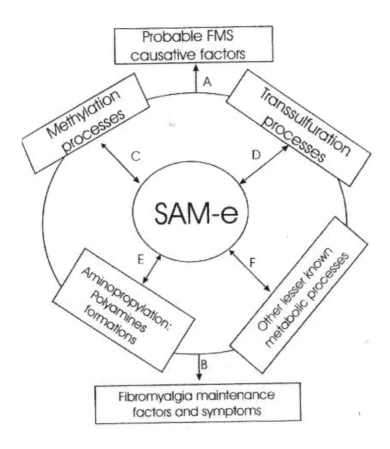

**Figure 10: A theoretical model for the probable action of SAM-e in the relief of fibromyalgia symptoms.**

B. Fibromyalgia maintenance factors and symptoms: Probable role of SAM e

- Depressive moods and fatigue
- Muscle pain and tender points
- Migraine headaches
- CNS sensory perception abnormalities
- Histamine and allergens
- Sleep or circadian rhythm disorders
- Too much oxidants and toxins in the body

C. Methylation processes

- Manufacture of neurotransmitters like dopamine, serotonin and melatonin
- DNA
- RNA
- Protein synthesis
- Phospholipid synthesis and regulation

D. Transsulfuration processes

- Gluthation formation and antioxidation
- Cysteine synthesis
- Taurin

E. Polyamines

Action of SAM e with arginine to catalyze the synthesis of

- Spermine
- Spermidine
- Putrescine

F. Several other lesser known metabolic processes in which SAM e acts as a precursor like:

- Propylamine component donation after decarboxylation
- As an allosteric factor in several conditions
- In bacterial DNA restriction and modification

•       Role in E. coli restriction and modification

•       Involved in the reduction of heavy metals like cobalt or iron in the process of transforming protein into a catalytically charged enzyme

•       Through transmethylation SAM e is intimately involved in the modulation of the different actions of norepinephrine and morphine

The healthcare implications of the above processes in which SAM e is involved are enormous. A complete discussion is far beyond the intended scope of this book.

SAM e and Gene Expression Abnormality

DNA (deoxyribonucleic acid) is the genetic blueprint of all living organisms. It is found in loosely coiled threads or helixes called chromatin, which aggregate to form chromosomes. RNAs, mRNA and tRNAs (ribonucleic acid, messenger RNA and transfer RNA) are responsible for the sequencing of amino acids in the formation of different protein compounds.

SAM e, through its methylation of DNA and RNA, activates or deactivates genes, which results in their growth and repair. This process has some implications on SAM e's action in cartilage formation and repair in osteoarthritis.

Activated genes also produce disease-fighting antibodies or regress tumors by gene deactivation. Therefore, an increase in SAM e levels in the system of fibromyalgia victims would promote faulty gene repair, cell health and action.

Also, SAM e has an important role in the manufacture of polyamines. These molecules contain nitrogen and are intimately involved with DNA and gene expression repairs.

SAM e and Sleep Disorders

Through methylation, SAM e reacts with serotonin to manufacture melatonin. Secreted by the pineal gland, melatonin is responsible for synchronizing hormonal release. It therefore regulates the so-called "circadian rhythm." Daylight acts as a precursor for the release of melatonin, and darkness suppresses its release. There is enough scientific evidence that shows that an imbalance in the melatonin production would result in insomnia and other sleep disorders.

A theory about aging, according to Dr. Julian Whitaker, is that the body is genetically programmed to wind down like a clock. Thus the balance between daytime and nighttime patterns gets blurred with age. Supplementing with melatonin, according to the doctor, would put "the tick and tock back into your ticktocks." But you won't need to, if you have optimal methylation.

The above would also have far-reaching effects on muscle soreness and fatigue experienced by fibromyalgia sufferers resulting from lack of restorative sleep. You see, our bodies are wired up like an electrical circuit; disconnect it at one spot, and the whole system shuts off.

Another research study worthy of mention is the one conducted in Germany by Offenbacher and associates titled: Possible association of fibromyalgia with a polymorphism in the serotonin transporter gene regulatory region. The method used was to analyze genomic DNA from 62 patients who have FMS per the American College of Rheumatology's diagnostic criteria. They also analyzed 110 healthy patients to act as controls. The study found a gene abnormality in fibromyalgia patients which resulted in altered serotonin metabolism. Serotonin is the precursor of melatonin.

SAM e, Abnormal Brain Function and Neurotransmitter Regulation

Several studies claim that toxic substances and metabolites associated with psychiatric disorders arise from a faulty transmethylation process of brain compounds also known as neurotransmitters. But further studies have narrowed down the problem to a failure of the transmethylation process. This, of course, would have implications for the role of SAM e in neurotransmitter methylation.

Neurotransmitters that are known to benefit from SAM e's activity include serotonin, epinephrine, norepinephrine and dopamine. The brain and the whole central nervous system would benefit from SAM e's phospholipid production, like phosphatidylserine. Lecithin is a supplementary phospholipid form. So proper supplementation with SAM e by fibromyalgia sufferers and the aged will definitely boost brain phospholipid production.

SAM e and High CSF Homocysteine Levels

Homocysteine, as I have already mentioned, maintains a seesaw relationship with SAM e. A very high level of homocysteine in the cerebrospinal fluid is a certain indication of low levels of SAM e in the body. Homocysteine, a sulfur-containing compound, can be beneficial in small amounts. Large amounts, however, lead to several diseases that include heart disease, cancer, depression and fibromyalgia. A Swedish study discovered a consistent connection between high levels of homocysteine and low levels of Vitamin B12 in cerebrospinal fluid (CSF) of fibromyalgia sufferers.

SAM e and Autoimmune Disorder

Faulty immune system activation results in excessive productions of immunoglobulins. According to David E. Berg and associates at the ITEMEX Laboratories in Phoenix, Arizona, every chronic fatigue syndrome and fibromyalgia patient they had ever worked with could trace onset to some previous disease state.

According to their research presented at the 1998 American Association of Chronic Fatigue Syndrome Conference in Cambridge, Massachusetts, the immunoglobulins poke holes through protective protein sheaths inside blood vessels. Consequently, excess thrombin converts fibrinogen into soluble fibrin monomer called fibrin.

The coating of the interior lining of these blood vessels blocks normal blood flow of essential oxygen and nutrients, thereby preventing surrounding body tissues from getting them.

SAM e, through DNA and RNA methylation, has repairing effects on this and other autoimmune problems.

SAM e, Depressive Moods and Fatigue

There is still some controversy whether fibromyalgia is caused by depression or psychiatric states, or whether fibromyalgia brings about depressions. Most likely, sufferers become depressed by the constant pain and low quality of life. There is both mental and physical fatigue due to poor unrestorative sleep. Other known causes of depression include:

- Serotonin deficiency
- Hormonal system imbalance
- Thyroid gland underactivity
- Deficiency of amino acids

- Nutritional deficiency
- Weakened immune system
- Environmental allergies and food sensitivities
- Poor stress-coping ability
- Too much toxins and oxidants in the body
- Inactivity and general deconditioning
- Inadequate light
- Stressful relationships
- Low blood sugar or hypoglycemia
- Lifestyle issues

Already, SAM e has been shown to regulate the action of many of the above-mentioned causative factors of depression. There is an overwhelming amount of scientific evidence that SAM e indeed would relieve depression even faster and better than regular antidepressants, without leaving behind the usual side effects.

According to the well-known expert in this matter, Dr. Richard Brown, SAM e is a powerful antidepressant which works gently in the body without the side effects of regular prescription drugs.

A study in 1973 in Verona, Italy gave SAM e to 20 depressed patients for 15 days; 10 were given only placebos. Using appropriate testing tools, the study found that the SAM e group showed some improvements in depressive moods, including attitude to work, among others. The researchers noted the rapid action of SAM e in treating depressive symptoms in as little as 4 to 7 days and with no side effects.

With regard to fibromyalgia depressive moods, some people have blamed biochemical imbalances, such as low levels of serotonin. This will eventually result in lack of restorative sleep, poor muscle micro-trauma repair and more pain.

A comparison of the effects of SAM e with those of regular antidepressants would show the following:

- SAM e is quicker, as soon as 4 to 7 days
- Leaves no real side effects, even in large doses
- Non-toxic
- Don't need to stop taking SAM e, since older persons may need to supplement anyway

SAM e, Muscle Pain and Tender Points

Clinical trials involving over 22,000 patients all found SAM e as effective in relieving muscle pain as NSAIDs (non-steroidal anti-inflammatory drugs), without leaving their side effects. A recent news report indicated that as many as 103,000 patients are hospitalized annually due to the serious gastric side effects of NSAIDs. About 16,500 fatalities are reported from this problem.

A study reported in the Current Therapeutic Research journal by Dr. P. DiBenedetto and colleagues compared SAM e with TENS (transcutaneous electrical nerve stimulation) on 30 fibromyalgia patients over a 6-week period. In the study, 15 patients received 200 mg of SAM e injection in the morning, with additional 200 mg tablets at noon and in the evening.

Another 15 persons only received TENS units to wear. All were tested using appropriate scales at the end of study. The study found that SAM e, when compared with TENS usage, reduced more tender points and had a significant beneficial effect on symptoms such as pain and fatigue. As regards depression, the

SAM e group showed reduced scores on the Hamilton Depression and Anxiety Rating Scales and also Zung's self-rating scale for depression.

Another process through which SAM e exerts its effects on pain is the process called aminopropylation. It is a process in which the polyamines spermidine and spermine are formed. These have important roles in tissue and cell growth. Another byproduct of this process is a compound called methylthioadenosine (MTA), which is known to be a player in the body's regulation of pain and inflammatory processes.

SAM e and Migraine Headaches

According to SAM e researcher Dr. Dallas Clouatre, SAM e is known to have beneficial effects for migraine headaches. According to him, the mechanism is not properly known, but may be due to an improvement in membrane fluidity and catecholamine balance regulation.

SAM e's Role in Controlling System Levels of Toxins, Oxidants, Histamine and Allergens

SAM e is able to regulate levels of toxins and other harmful metabolites in the system by influencing the production of the body's primary antioxidant and free-radical scavenger called glutathione. Free radicals are byproducts of glycolysis that are harmful to the body and may be involved with the problem of fibromyalgia. Another antioxidant is taurin, which also results from the process of transsulfuration.

Asthma, allergies and other disease conditions, including fibromyalgia, may be worsened or maintained by histamines in the body. Histamine is set off when organs that are exposed to the environment, like skin and the respiratory tract, get in contact with substances called allergens. The body regulates the amount of histamine in the body through an enzyme called histamine N-methyltransferase (HMT). This enzyme, according to biochemist Dr. Cooney, requires SAM e as a methyl donor. This makes SAM e an important player in histamine level regulation.

Other Recent Scientific Studies on the Effects of SAM E on Fibromyalgia

Italy 1987: Evaluation of SAM e in primary fibromyalgia. A double-blind cross-over study. Conducted by Dr. A. Tavoni and associates.

Method used: 17 people with fibromyalgia took part in a scientific investigation in which a group receives one form of treatment before "crossing over" to get another type. Group A received 200 mg of SAM e daily and orally, while Group B received what looked like SAM e but was not (placebo). After 21 days both groups stopped taking anything. They were given 14 days to cool off. Why? So that whatever each group took will wear off.

Then after 14 days, both groups switched places. When the results were tallied, the researchers found a significant amount of improvement in the moods and fewer numbers of painful sites and tender points in the SAM e group (Group A) than the placebo group (Group B). Because of this, those doctors decided that SAM e is indeed effective in treating primary fibromyalgia.

Denmark 1991: Oral SAM e in primary fibromyalgia. Double-blind clinical evaluation. Conducted by Dr. Jacobsen and associates. Reported in the Scandinavian Journal of Rheumatology.

Method: 44 fibromyalgia patients participated. Twenty received 800 mg of SAM e daily and orally. The other group of 20 received just placebo. It is called double-blind since nobody knew what they actually received, whether the real thing or a tablet that looked like SAM e but was not. After the 6 weeks of the study, the investigators reported an improvement in fibromyalgia symptoms of fatigue, pain, morning stiffness and mood in the SAM e group when compared to placebo group.

Italy 1994: Primary fibromyalgia is responsive to SAM e. Conducted by Drs. Grassetto and Varotto. Reported in Current Therapeutic Research.

Method: 47 fibromyalgia patients were treated with 200 mg of SAM e given intramuscularly once daily and 400 mg taken twice (800 mg) daily for 6 weeks. Researchers found at the end of study that SAM e had improved participants' fibromyalgia symptoms of tender points, depressive moods and anxiety.

The overall verdict on SAM e's performance was that it was an effective remedy for depressed moods, pain and general well-being. And since poor sleep is a by-product of pain, SAM e would also be beneficial in improving sleep quality.

United States 1994: SAM e in Sjögren's syndrome and fibromyalgia.

Method: 30 patients with Sjögren's syndrome, fibromyalgia or both were treated with 200 mg of SAM e given by intramuscular injection. All patients showed some improvements in their depression and for the fibromyalgia-only participants, there was a significant improvement and reduction in number of painful sites.

# Chapter 11: Other Uses Of SAMe?

As we have already discussed, SAM e is able to effect and modulate several of our bodies' metabolic processes due to its readiness to donate its reactive methyl group to several receptor molecules to form new compounds. SAM e, through methylation, transsulfuration and a host of other lesser-known processes, is able to maintain our bodies in optimal health. It can also repair the damage done and alleviate symptoms of other disease states such as

- Osteoarthritis
- Liver diseases
- Brain diseases such as Parkinson's and Alzheimer's
- Cardiovascular diseases
- Many others

SAM e and Osteoarthritis

Osteoarthritis is a degenerative joint disease that affects millions of Americans. It attacks the normally smooth joint surfaces of our bones. Cracks and fissures develop. Weight-bearing stresses worsen condition. In time, the synovial fluid, which lubricates the joint surfaces, dries up or leaks into the fissures and cracks, then into the bone. Gradually blood vessels grow out of these cracks, into joint gaps which they occlude. Osteophytes or bony outgrowths form and end up restricting joint motion. By this time, the joint is usually swollen and very painful.

The usual treatment of choice is NSAIDs – non-steroidal anti-inflammatory drugs and other pain medications. These drugs have been known to cause adverse reactions such as protein breakdown and can inhibit cartilage formation and proteoglycan synthesis. Other problems of long-term use of NSAIDs include serious gastric problems.

SAM e provides comparable relief to arthritis pain when compared to NSAIDs, but without any side effects. Also, SAM e appears to promote native proteoglycan synthesis, which are important factors in cartilage repair.

SAM e additionally may provide gastric cytoprotection against aspirin-induced hemorrhagic erosions, probably due to its ability to assist in glutathione production and its ability to protect the intestinal lining from the attacks of toxins.

SAM e and the Liver

The liver is one of the most important and largest organs in the body. It controls processes that help sustain life; processes fats, removes toxins, produces the all-important bile. SAM e is known to assist in many of the liver's functions and protects it from harmful toxins. SAM e, for example, through methylation, converts phosphatidylethanolamine into phosphatidylcholine, a useful lipotropic.

In liver cirrhosis, an essential enzyme for SAM e's product may be lacking. The disease appears to restrict "SAM e synthetase," which results in impaired SAM e production. Consequently, methionine, the building block of SAM e, is not utilized. High quantities of this substance can become harmful to the liver. Because of this problem, it would be a good idea to supplement with pharmaceutical SAM e, thereby bypassing this production impasse. This would enable SAM e to continue to function in the liver. SAM e is important in the liver's ability to make bile salts.

Without bile salts, the liver is unable to digest fats and consequently other of its functions will be stalled.

SAM e and Brain Diseases like Parkinson's and Alzheimer's

As part of the aging process, there is a decline of methylation in the brain, which may have some implications with the disease progress of Parkinson's and Alzheimer's.

Parkinson's disease is a degenerative problem affecting an area of the mid-brain known as the substantia nigra. This is an area whose job is to produce dopamine, which is a very important neurotransmitter. SAM e's role in Parkinson's disease is not very clear. Actually, some people believe that high levels of SAM e may be detrimental for this condition.

The problem of Alzheimer's is a progressive diminishing of cognitive functions in areas of short-term memory; they have spatial problems and an inability to remember things or persons. They can sometimes behave in inappropriate or even bizarre manners.

SAM e's role in Alzheimer's is not well known by the research community. What they know, however, is that SAM e levels are severely decreased in these patients when compared to normal subjects. Some interpret this as a supply and demand situation, i.e., excessive need for SAM e, which the aging brain is unable to supply. This argument is buttressed by the fact that some memory function improvements can be achieved with SAM e supplementation in some cases.

SAM e and Cardiovascular Diseases

Cardiovascular disease affects the blood vessels and the coronary arteries of the heart. The commonest condition is atherosclerosis. This is the blocking of the arteries by a combination of fatty substances, cholesterol and other wastes. A person is said to suffer a heart attack when the occlusion of a heart artery shuts off blood supply to the heart. Common risk factors include cigarette smoking, high cholesterol levels, diabetes and inactivity.

SAM e's role in heart disease is with controlling the levels of homocysteine, a well-known culprit in heart diseases. Homocysteine allegedly promotes the accumulation of waste in the inner lining of blood vessels by irritation of those linings; it can also prevent the vessels from dilating sufficiently.

In a normal system, homocysteine is a normal by-product of methylation and transsulfuration. Deficiencies of nutrients like folic acid, Vitamin B12 and Vitamin B6 have been known to impair normal methylation and transsulfurization processes. So these supplements should be taken along with SAM e.

# Chapter 12: How To Take SAMe For Fibromyalgia

I have heard some people complain that SAM e didn't seem to work for them even after one week of taking it. There may be various reasons for this. Questions you can ask yourself about the SAM e you are taking are:

• Did you take SAM e at all? SAM e is so unstable that if not packaged and stored properly, its potency will quickly disappear.

• Was your SAM e up to standard? Were you sure that what was claimed on the label was actually what was inside the bottle? Remember the FDA does not regulate the manufacture and distribution of SAM e as it does prescription drugs. So you really are responsible for making sure you purchase the right SAM e.

• Did you take enough dosage of SAM e? And how did you take it? With vodka? On empty or full stomach? These things do matter a lot.

Dosage would depend on your condition and its severity. But SAM e is quite safe. Your main limitation, as I suspect, might be the size of your wallet. Presently, SAM e is very expensive.

The following are some of what is known about pharmaceutical grade SAM e.

The amount of SAM e that eventually enters your bloodstream and the length of time it takes to get there would depend on the following factors:

- Its ability to remain in one piece until it reaches your bloodstream
- How fast the liver metabolizes it and how quickly your kidney excretes it
- The higher the dosage and the higher its staying power would be

The length of time it takes a certain quantity of SAM e to get to half of its original quantity in the blood is known as its half-life. That is, if it takes 3 hours for 200 mg of SAM e to get to 100 mg, the half-life is 3 hours. Researchers have put SAM e's half-life to about 101 minutes for a dosage of 500 mg.

Rate of SAM e absorption is fastest with intravenous administration. The slowest is oral administration. The advantage of this method is that it will act for a longer period. The optimal absorption of SAM e is achieved in the intestines and not in the stomach. So to allow it to get past the stomach/s digestive environment, SAM e should be taken in an enteric-coated form. SAM e is best absorbed when taken on an empty stomach.

TOXICITY

There is no evidence of its toxicity in humans. In rats, an ingestion of 1200 mg per kg for about 30 days did not produce any adverse symptoms, and it did not upset the digestive system. This is perhaps one of the reasons SAM e should be preferred over NSAIDs, especially in osteoporosis. In osteoporosis, unlike the NSAIDs, which are notorious for impeding cartilage damage repair, SAM e actually helps produce a cartilage-repairing protein called proteoglycan.

## DOSAGE

Some experts recommend a dosage of 200 mg to 400 mg of enteric-coated SAM e two times a day. That is a total of up to 800 mg daily.

## POSSIBLE SIDE EFFECTS

Not much. Some clinical studies have reported some mild gastrointestinal upsets and nausea in some people, especially at very high doses. If this becomes a problem for you, start with small doses and progress until you achieve your own optimal dosage. You can also do a large dose in small single doses spread out through the day.

## CONTRAINDICATIONS

Methionine may be harmful to menopausal and postmenopausal women, please use with care. If you have manic psychological illness, please discuss with your psychiatrist before using SAM e. Some clinical studies suggest SAM e may be contraindicated for manic-depressive states.

## OPTIMAL DOSAGE RECOMMENDATION

This is only a guideline. Talk to your doctor, especially if you plan to stop your addictive medications. I am not aware of any reported drug interaction problems with SAM e.

For fibromyalgia with depressive moods

Take 400 mg of SAM e 3 to 4 times daily (maximum 1600 mg)

Start with 200 mg 2x daily for day #1

Increase to 400 mg 2x daily by day #3

Increase to 400 mg 3x daily by day #10

Get to maximum dosage of 400 mg 4x daily after 20 days and continue as needed.

If you need SAM e for regular supplementation to boost your body's methylation system, 200 mg 2 to 3x daily might be sufficient.

OSTEOARTHRITIS

Use the same method outlined above for fibromyalgia. Max out at 400 mg 3x daily on day #10, continue at this dosage for another 10 days or more as needed. After about one month at maximum dosage, you might want to reduce to a maintenance dose of 200 mg 2x daily.

LIVER DISORDERS

200 mg to 400 mg 2 to 3x daily

MIGRAINE HEADACHES

200 mg to 400 mg 2 to 3x daily

DEPRESSION

Use same exact method as for fibromyalgia with depressive symptoms.

# Chapter 13: Ideas About How To Safely Come Off Your Addictive Medications

Your life with fibromyalgia syndrome may be likened to a ship caught in a stormy sea – the sea of pain and you are supposed to be the captain. But are you really the captain of your life or have you given over command to someone else? Perhaps your doctor. Too much medication may have immobilized this captain. It is very important that you remain in charge. After all, it is still your life, not anyone else's.

Some people buy into some myths about our country's current healthcare situation. Myths like:
- My doctor knows best, whatever he prescribes is fine.
- If the FDA approved it, it must be good.
- I heard it on TV, many people are taking it, therefore, it must be good.

All the above are false assumptions. Your doctor may mean well, but he is a pawn within the managed care game. Besides, he may be the product of a conventional mindset about treating fibromyalgia symptoms, while ignoring the underlying problems, like lifestyle options and choices, bad habits, relationship issues, spirituality and a host of other predisposing factors. Some of these factors were not usually taught in the basic medical training, although that problem may now be changing with the current general public fascination with alternative or integrative medicine.

The second myth is about the FDA and the drug approval process. The FDA may not be all that impartial watchdog, it is purported to be. Powerful drug companies and other interest groups, may be holding the leash from behind the scenes.

The drug companies, court medical students right up to graduation and beyond, with public relation gifts and incentive offers. Doctors' offices are full of Public Relations items and drug samples. The drug companies fund medical studies, sponsor seminars the doctors must attend in order to maintain their certifications. They keep research journals in business by maintaining huge advertisement accounts.

One way or the other they try to influence what is being published. Recently, a drug company threatened to full its huge advertisement account with a reputable medical journal, simply because a study that was detrimental to one of its products was published.

Furthermore, TV talk shows may not be the citadel of wisdom some people think it is. This is because the producer's main concern is sensationalism. Every program is about rating and turning huge profits. Then they promote the quick fixes for every human problem, usually in pill bottles. But there are no quick fixes. Our lifestyle is a product of ten of a lifetime of bad choices, so solutions will take time.

Sometime the medications are necessary, but we must watch out for ourselves. There are adverse reactions, addiction problems, withdrawal reaction problems, drug interaction problems and so many others. The so-called beneficial medications cause as much as 140,000 fatalities annually. We ought to reconsider our quick fix pill-popping mindset and consider altering our lifestyle.

Alternatives to Antidepressants

- Learn to cope with stress and tension.
- Learn and practice "Muscle Tension Relaxation technique," which I will explain                later.
- Organize and manage your life better.
- Control your worry and anxiety before it controls you.
- Build-up self-confidence and self-esteem.
- Establish a restorative sleep hygiene.
- Confront your nagging fears.
- Learn to be more assertive.
- Let your friends and relatives know your limitations and boundaries.
- Resolve relationship problems quickly, forgive and move on.
- Let go of the past and learn to forgive.
- Be focused and keep things in their proper perspective.
- Above all, pray as if everything depends on God, and act as if everything depends on                you.

Ideas on How to Come Off or Decrease the Dosage of Your Addictive Medications

According to specialists in this field like Drs. Peter Breggin and David Cohen, the best and most sensible method, is a gradual and well-planned one. According to these experts "regardless of the drug you are using and the problems it may have created in your life, a well-planned, gradual withdrawal has the best chance to succeed." On the other hand, an unplanned on-the-spur-of the moment decision would only cause more problems and frustration.

It is crucial that you are convinced in what you plan to do. Place before you always, the many benefits you are hoping to achieve. List the difficulties you might encounter and expect them. Expect possible relapses. It is okay, you can always try again.

Find a psychiatrist who believes in what you plan to do, and is willing to support you. Keep company with people who are likely to encourage you in your resolution. Expect that some people will be negative about it. If it didn't work for them, it won't work for you, they would suggest. Don't let their fears and lack of self-confidence rub off on you. But whatever happens, be in control of the situation, it is still your body and life.

The adverse reactions you may encounter would not mean you "really need this medication." It is only what is called "withdrawal reactions." Don't be discouraged.

Pray. God, they say, helps those who help themselves. Find a support group of relatives and friends. Find a supporter, willing to speak with you often. Involve your spouse and family members. The will and enthusiasm to live fully and to take back your life from fibromyalgia, will soon rub off on these around you, and they will appreciate you more. Check out the information super highway – the Internet for encouraging websites.

A Step-by-Step Gradual Drug Withdrawal Plan

Step 1:    Stabilize your dose by taking the same amount, same time.

Step 2:    Choose a gradual stepwise method, like reducing dose by 10% or any other amount you          are      comfortable with. You may start with the SAM-e program to coincide with this.    This would cushion the normal withdrawal reactions.

In the 10% technique, you are supposed to decrease your dosage in ten steps, 10% at a time. You may divide the last dose into smaller doses.

The duration of each step would depend on how long you've been on that medication. This is the Law of Habit at play. It took some time building an addiction, dismantling that habit would also take time. In general, it may vary from weeks to months. You are in charge here. Make a plan and stick with it; at the same time expand your alternative medicine strategies.

For example, if you are taking 150 mg of an anti-depressant, your first cut (decrease) would be 15mg. Perform the next eight 15 mg cuts, then you can subdivide the last or tenth 15 mg, into smaller cuts if you prefer. Stay on each step for one week to ten days. The last step is usually the toughest, that is why you might have to subdivide it.

What to Do About Withdrawal Reactions

1. It is hoped that supplementing with SAM-e will help a great deal with this problem.

2.  Depending on how long you've been on medication, you might have to do very small cuts, less than 10%, and remain in each step for longer periods.

3.  If you are on several drugs, plan to stop one at a time. Start with the heavy ones; i.e., if you are taking one to relieve the side-effects of the other, then remove the side-effect medication later.

4.  You may have to cool off for a long time after decreasing to a lower dose. Adjust to the reactions, before venturing again, but try not to despair or discard the whole idea. You have one life to live, you will not have another chance. Think of all those who love you and need you to be strong and together. For the Christian believer, the words of Christ to Paul the apostle suffices, "My grace is sufficient for you." You just have to pray to tap into this reservoir of strength.

# Chapter 14: How To Manage Stress And Muscle Tension

**What is Stress?**

Life is naturally stressful. Our bodies are made up of chemicals and hormones that are constantly at war with each other. We live on a high-tech and high pressure society which is a maelstrom of all kinds of stressors.

We can't always get what we want. We clutter our lives with things we don't need. Then we have fragile egos that get in the way of meaningful relationships. We get caught up in bad habits that dill us gradually. The changes we can make, we are reluctant in making, the ones we can't, we worry needlessly over. We entertain irrational fears over things we can't control. So, we are enveloped by stressors, which gradually master our lives.

Science defines acute stress as a reaction to an immediate danger. This is also called the "fight or flight" response. What this means in layman's terms is that nature automatically prepares us to face danger. Our hearts beat faster and pump more blood and oxygen to the muscles where there might be needed to affect an escape or to ut up a fight. Many other things happen within our bodies.

This beneficial protective reaction can become habitual. When this happens, our bodies re-adjust in a very wrong way. A sense of tension resides in our subconscious and continually feed our senses with undesirable stimuli. Our tension senses become lowered and so every little, harmless event puts our bodies in "red alert." Somehow the physiological changes that occur when we are faced with a threat do not go back to normal anymore. This situation is known as residual tension.

What is Muscle Tension?

There are two connotations to the term "muscle tension."

- Muscle fibers are contracting needlessly, even when subject is at rest.

- There is a constant tension sense. Muscles remain in a shortened position.

The following are some clinical evidence of a state of muscle tension:

- Irregular and shallow breathing.

- Your mind is as busy as a beehive when you are supposed to be sleeping.

- Your brow frowns and your eyelids move uncontrollably.

- Any little thing startles you.

- There is spasm of the smooth muscles of the alimentary canal.

- You can't sleep at night, you jerk and toss around.

What are the Noticeable Signs of Stress?

- You get upset easily.

- You worry too much.

- You forget thing and you can't concentrate.

- You procrastinate.

- You can't seem to keep appointments or manage your time well.

- You start taking tranquilizers.

- Because of poor sleep quality, your muscles are always sore.

The Short-Term Effects of Stress, i.e., "The Fight or Flight" Response

Each stressful episode starts a chain reaction in your system:

Large quantities of epinephrine is released into your bloodstream.

Your heart beats faster.

Your blood pressure rises.

Your breathing becomes faster and shallow.

Your metabolic rate escalates.

Muscle tension rises with increased lactic acid.

Your blood gets re-routed to your muscles away from the digestive system.

This causes an imbalance in the digestive juices and they start chopping away at your stomach lining causing ulcers.

Cortisol decreases your immune system, and so you easily get sick and have frequent flu and fevers.

Long-Term Effects of Stress

If you do nothing about how you react to stress and you live a habitual life of stress and tension, gradually, your body adjusts and produce more serious symptoms like:

- High blood pressure
- Frequent headaches
- Sleep problems

- You become easily irritable.
- You will develop high cholesterol levels which eventually will clog your arteries.
- You always struggle to catch your breath with little exertion.
- Palpitations of the heart; perhaps develop abnormal heart rhythms.
- Muscle and back pain due to decreased blood flow of nutrients and oxygen; accumulation of metabolites like lactic acid.
- Nausea: unpleasant sensation in the stomach caused by gastric acid production imbalance.
- Ulcers develop.
- Production of too much Cortisol which decreases your immune system resulting in frequent illnesses.
- Depressive moods.

What is Relaxation?

Now we understand the serious problems caused by stress, we now turn our attention to its exact opposite – Relaxation. Relaxation provokes opposite physiological reactions to those of stress, some of these include:

- Decreased epinephmine in the blood, this leads to lowering of blood pressures, with less stress on the cardiovascular system.
- Less clogging of arteries due to reduced blood sugar and cholesterol. Risk of heart attacks is reduced significantly.

- Breathing is slower and deeper. More oxygen and nutrients get to the brain and the muscles. This improves metabolic rate.

- Quality of sleep will improve, allowing the secretion of repairing hormones from the pituitary gland.

- There is improved digestion. No ulcers, which allows you to enjoy all kinds of food.

- The immune system remains in top shape, and you become less prone to illnesses.

The overall effect of relaxation is a regular state of serenity, with increased alertness and spontaneity. So the state of relaxation is a very desirable one especially for the fibromyalgia sufferer. It doesn't come easy. It is a skill to be learned. When learned and practiced regularly, soon becomes second nature. This Science of Relaxation is called Progressive Muscle Relaxation. Once you master the art of relaxation, you won't ever need tranquilizers to calm down. You will learn to relax beyond the residual tension state.

What Happens in "Physiological" Relaxation?

- There is complete absence of muscle contraction.
- Muscle fibers remain in a lengthen position.
- The big skeletal muscles become limp.
- Rate of impulse firing, and excitability of nerves become reduced or even inactive.

Progressive Relaxation Technique

There are several types of this technique. It is better to just learn and master one technique. Relaxation is Relaxation, it doesn't really matter how you become relaxed. First described as a science by Dr. Edmund Jacobson in 1908, followed by other investigators of this phenomenon including Dr. Herbert Benson. In 1970, Dr. Benson wrote his definitive book on the subject called "The Relaxation Response." This is basically the opposite of the "fight or flight" response to a treat or a stressful event.

How Much Time Do You Need?

Researchers found that a 20-minute practice each day was very beneficial to both physical and mental health.

What You Need to Induce a Relaxation Response

- Quiet environment
- A comfortable position
- A point of focus
- A passive attitude

Most people always manage to make out time for things that they consider important, like favorite talk show schedules. So try and make time for relaxation. It may very well make the difference between life and death. And it would certainly improve and prolong your life.

Breathing Exercise

Some of the benefits of biofeedback therapy include helping you become aware of subtle muscle activity you are not ordinarily conscious of; use your muscles better. It teaches you breathing skills to encourage muscle tension release and physiologic quieting.

Improper and shallow breathing habit prevents your muscles from getting the oxygen and nutrients they need. It is therefore important to re-learn how to breathe properly. A common method is called diaphragmatic breathing technique.

Technique

Sit comfortably like in Figure 14-1.

Joseph K. Egbebike, PhD.,PT

Write notes here:

# Figure 14-1 Diaphragmatic Breathing Technique

**Figure 14-1: Diaphragmatic Breathing Technique**

A. Sit comfortably as shown. Place both of your hands on your stomach just below the rib cage. Breathe in gradually and deeply through the nose. Allow your diaphragm to move down and flatten as your stomach moves forward pushing out your hands. Feel your fingers fan out.

B. Hold your breath for about 5 seconds and gradually breathe out through the nose. Feel your diaphragm relax and your stomach sink. Try to let out as much air as possible.

C. Repeat this procedure 3 to 4 times. Focus your mind on this exercise; avoid all distractions. Your chest is supposed to remain still during this exercise. If it moves, you may be doing it incorrectly.

D. Practice with your spouse (see below). Everybody needs it to relax completely; your spouse probably needs it more than you do! Besides, it is a nice way of communicating and getting involved.

**Figure 14-2: Two-Person Breathing Technique**

Assume position as in Figure 14-2. Place your hands in the shape of a "V" below your spouse's rib cage. Ask him or her to breathe in slowly, allowing the stomach to rise. Make sure your spouse's chest is not moving. Feel his or her stomach pushing out your hands. Then ask your spouse to slowly let out air through the nose. Repeat 3 to 4 times. Switch positions and repeat the procedure.

A. Place both of your hands on your tummy just below the rib cage. Breathe in gradually and deeply through the nose. Allow your diaphragm to move down and flatten, as your stomach moves forward pushing out your hands. Feel your fingers fan out.

B. Hold your breath for about 5 seconds and gradually breathe out through the nose. Feel your diaphragm relax and your stomach sink. Try to let out, as much air as possible.

C. Repeat this procedure about 3 to 4 times. Focus your mind on this exercise, avoid all distractions. Your chest is supposed to remain still during this exercise, otherwise you may be doing it wrongly.

D.Practice together with your spouse. Everybody needs it to relax completely. And your spouse probably needs it more than you do; and besides, it is a nice way of communicating and getting involved.

Assume position as in Figure 14-2.

Figure 14-2 Two persons breathing technique practice.

Place both of your hands in a "V" shaped form below his rib cage. Ask him to breathe in slowly allowing his stomach to rise. Make sure his chest is not moving also. Feel his stomach push out your hands. Then ask him to slowly let out air through the nose. Repeat 3 to 4 times. Exchange positions and repeat procedure.

Progressive Muscle Relaxation Technique

As mentioned earlier on, you will need the following:

- A quiet environment
- Comfortable position
- A point of focus
- A passive attitude

Step 1. Quiet Environment

This is difficult to find or arrange when you have children. But you must find one. Be creative, negotiate if you must. Place "don't disturb signs" on doors; sneak down to the basement. Just find the space and do it!

Step 2. A Comfortable Position

Depending on what your goal is, assume position of figure 14-3 (Lying down), if you intend to sleep off, or position of figure 14-4 (sitting or reclining).

Figure 14-3: Relaxation Position: Lying Down

Place pillows under the head and knees, place arms loosely at your sides with the palm flat on the mattress. You should feel completely relaxed. This position is called "the Neutral position." Tension is zero.

**Figure 14-3: Relaxation Position: Lying Down**
Place pillows under the head and knees, lay arms loosely at your sides with the palms face down on the mattress. You should feel completely relaxed. This position is called "the neutral position." Tension is zero.

**Figure 14-4: Relaxation Position: Sitting Down**
Sit comfortably in a high-backed chair that supports your head and whole spine. Place both arms tension-free on the armrests as shown.

Figure 14-4 Relaxation Position: Sitting Down

Sit comfortable in a high-backed chair that supports your head and whole spine. Place both arms tension-free on the arm-rests as shown.

You can also sit straight (as in figure 14-1) with a straight spine or you can sit cross-legged.

### Step 3. A point of focus

Choose a special word of phrase, and repeat throughout the session. This is very similar to the Christian form of meditation called the "Jesus Prayer" and in fact is used as a relaxation prayer. It goes like this: "Jesus, Son of the living God, have mercy on me, a sinner" or "The Lord is my Shepherd, I shall not want." You ca n practice with eyes either open or closed. If open, try to focus on some object, otherwise your mind will wander with your eyes.

### Step 4. A passive attitude

Let it happen. Right now, in this place and time, you don't care about anything. Don't worry about any distracting thoughts, this is normal. Gently turn about your attention to your point of focus.

### Step 5. Progressive muscle relaxation

There are several methods, the best is whatever suits your personality. The point is to relax. You can't relax except you know what tension is, then you strive for the opposite situation. That is why you need to forcefully contract each group of large skeletal muscles before you attempt to relax them.

If you are experiencing pain and worry that contracting our muscles will exacerbate it, then don't contract. You already know what tension is, just relax consciously. Like you are deflating like an inflated object. Where you start from, is not really important. Although it is advisable to end with the head.

(A) Feet and Toes: Start with the toes and move up. Crunch your toes and circle your ankles, then release.

(B) Leg muscles: Move your ankles completely up and down, hold then release.

(C) Thigh muscles: If you are laying down, press down the back of your knee on a rolled towel or pillow and squeeze your thighs or quads. Hold and release if sitting, hook your feet under something and try to raise it, while squeezing thighs, hold and release.

(D) Your Buttocks: Squeeze them, hold and release.

(E) Your Stomach: Pull it in, hold and release.

(F) Shoulders and back: Shrug shoulder and pull backwards, hold and release. Again arch the back, hold and then release.

(G) Neck muscles: If you are sitting, place both hands behind your head and push head backwards against your hands' resistance, hold and then release.

If you are laying, stiffen the muscles of the neck, hold and then release.

(H) Arms and hands

Flex (Show-off) your biceps i.e. bend your elbows hold and release.

Make a tight firs, hold and relax.

(I)  Head and facial muscles

Wrinkle your forehead, hold and release.

Frown deeply, hold and release.

Move from pursing your lips to a wide grin, repeat and release.

(J)  Eyes: Close the eyes tightly. Look up while maintaining your head position, then relax the eyes. Look down and repeat procedure. Relaxing the eyes, brow or lids, needs a lot of practice.

If you are not able to relax the eyes, try doing that at the same time yo do same with right arm.

General Comments

1.      You can interspace with breathing exercise.

2.      Hold tension for about 10 to 15 seconds.

3.      You can release in three steps.

4.      You can breathe in as you contract and hold, and breathe out as you release.

5.      Rest for about 1 minute or more in between muscle groups.

6.      Tense and Release only one group of muscles at a time, Keep the rest of your body perfectly still and relaxed.

Visualization

Create your favorite picture of peace and serenity and stay there. If your worries come up again, gently notice them and go back to your peaceful place.

Aromatherapy

You can light your favorite aromatic candle and put on a gentle relaxation music or sound like singing birds, gentle rainfall, etc.

## How to Stop Worrying

Worry in general is a stream of thoughts of fear that an event might occur. Your mind is like a wild horse that you must tame. Set aside a worry-time, when you can dwell on finding resolutions for the source of worry.

I personally like to actually list strategies to prevent the event from occurring, then I reconcile myself to the worst case scenarios that it may happen. I even make contingency plans, in case it does happen. The ones I can't do anything about, I don't worry about. My religious faith assures me that a loving God is still in charge of His creation, in spite of the seeming chaos.

Dealing with Anger and Resentment

Anger really hurts the angry person. It can cause serious health complications like heart disease and ulcers. Most of the time, anger cannot be controlled. It may be an indication that we are stressed, and it is time to take a break.

You really need to work on your anger or resentment if it is habitually on your mind and upsetting your life.

–      If it makes you abusive towards others

–      If it is hurting your relationship with family members.

Quick Solutions to Anger

1.   Acknowledge that you are angry. If you don't, it will never go away.

2.   Tame your mind and force it to dwell on happy thoughts.

3.   Rationalize your anger. Perhaps you are over-reaching and may need to cool off.

4.   Identify your source of anger. Learn to delay responding to someone's annoying remarks, you can count about ten mentally. Be in control of your emotions. Silence is the best answer, they say.

5.   Learn to listen to the other person. You might learn something that will be to your advantage. Try to see things sometimes form the other person's perspective and be firm and assertive when you must, but do this kindly.

Relationships

It is the bed you make, that you lie on. If you put rocks in yours, you will either remove them and lie on them, and they will continue to hurt you until you remove them. No one can help you with this. If you choose to move to another bed, pretty soon you'll come to realize that most beds are basically the same. Then you will have to start all over learning how to lie on this new one. So it makes a lot of sense to take care of the old one you are used to. Except, of course, the old bed is something else.

The point is that little unresolved relationship issues can quickly add up and get out of hand. Move away from too much self-preoccupation and realize your spouse for example has feelings too. Appreciate his efforts to understand and support you with your life of pain. See an appropriate therapist to help you resolve difficult issues like sex. Your psychiatrist can perhaps change your antidepressants to those that do not impair libido.

Humans they say, are social beings. You can't be alone for too long and not pay for it in mental health. You need your friends and relatives to feel valued, important and loved. A huge ego is a handicap, it is not in your best interest. Be the first to call and mend a relationship. If you want to change others, start by changing yourself.

Find a support group and attend meetings. This is an opportunity to be with people who can effect you in your current situation in a very positive way. You can learn new remedies to your health problems, or learn about sources of help.

The Importance of Laughing

"We don't laugh because we're happy – we're happy because we laugh."

— William James, psychologist

Nothing deflates anger and sadness that laughter. If a friend or something provokes us to laughter, we soon realize the foolishness of our depressive moods. There is now a science that deals with humor and treatment of disease states called humor therapy. According to noted author Norman Cousins (Anatomy of An Illness), he had discovered that 10 minutes of vigorous laughing bought him 2 hours of good sleeping without drugs or pain. Some researchers believe that laughing stimulates the release of chemical messengers in the brain known as endorphins, which are natural sedatives.

After a bout of laughter, blood pressure monitoring usually shows a decrease in readings, breathing is slower and deeper and muscles more relaxed. If you don't find anything funny enough, go watch a good comedy movie. If that don't do it, watch yourself in a mirror and start laughing, pretty soon you will be laughing for real.

# Chapter 15: Fibromyalgia Exercise And Fitness Program

Movement is a major characteristic of all living organisms and lack of it has a very great impact on the quality of life itself. Lack of exercise, especially for a prolonged period of time, for whatever reasons, has very profound effects on human cardiovascular, neuromuscular and metabolic systems. These effects can occur very rapidly.

For over a decade, I worked with geriatric patients in nursing homes and was able to observe firsthand how rapidly the muscles could succumb to inactivity. Most elders end up losing their ability to walk and independence because of this. The adage that "if you don't use it, you'll lose it" holds very true for muscles. Some of the well-known effects of lack of exercise include:

• Low energy and work capacity due to low oxygen uptake and usage.

• The muscles decrease in size, leading to decreased strength.

• Decreased cardiac efficiency leading to a decrease in circulating blood, plasma and red blood cells. This leads to several kinds of heart diseases.

• Decreased amount of air in the lungs.

• Increased amount of calcium is excreted in urine, leading to osteoporosis and fractures.

These problems have a ripple effect as they quickly create other health complications. There having a very painful condition like fibromyalgia will not be enough excuse not to exercise. We must find ways to control the pain; pace ourselves, but seize all available opportunity to exercise to a target heart rate of 60% to 80% of your maximum heart rate for about 20 to 30 minutes a day, at least three times a week.

## Some Scientific Investigations About Fibromyalgia and Exercise

1. A study to determine the effectiveness of physical training in women with fibromyalgia.

Conducted by C.S. Burckhardt and others and reported in Journal of Rheumatology.

99 women with fibromyalgia participated in this study and were divided into three groups. First group received only advice on self-management, the second group received advice and physical training, while the third group served as a control only. The results showed that those in groups one and two had significant improvements in their quality of life as evidenced by a decrease in feeling of helplessness, tender points, depressive moods and physical dysfunction.

2. A study to determine the effects of cardiovascular fitness on fibromyalgia.

G.A. McCain, D.A. Bell and associates. Studies were reported in the Arthritis and Rheumatology Journal.

42 patients with fibromyalgia were split into two groups and participated in this research program for 20 weeks. One group received cardiovascular fitness (CVR), the other group received only

simple flexibility exercises (FLEX) that did not promote cardio-vascular fitness. The exercise was for one hour, three times each week.

The results showed significant improvement in cardiovas-cular fitness scores in the CVR group, more than the FLEX group. Furthermore, the CVR group also showed significant im-provements in pain threshold values.

There are several other studies that show good evidence about the beneficial effects of exercise and fitness training on fi-bromyalgia. The major salient points to be deduced from these studies include:

- Exercise improves pain of fibromyalgia.
- It alleviates depressive moods.
- It improves cardiovascular health.
- Cardiovascular fitness requires aerobic activity.
- Fibromyalgia patients can include aerobic, flexibil-ity and strength training exercise without adverse effects.

According to Dr. George W. Waylonis, a professor of physical medicine and rehabilitation at Ohio State University: "The most effective treatments for fibromyalgia are exercise, over-the-counter pain medications and avoidance of stress fac-tors." According to several clinical studies, fibromyalgia patients are generally de-conditioned, and so a well-tailored exercise pro-gram is the hallmark of an adequate treatment program.

## Exercise Guidelines for Fibromyalgia

According to Dr. Russel, director of the Clinical Research Center at the University of Texas Health Science Center in San

Antonio, fibromyalgia exercise and fitness programs should be started slowly, and progressed gradually according to the patient's tolerance. He points out that "unaccustomed physical exertion can induce severe body pain and incapacitate the patient for the next several days."

•        Patient should get a medical check-up for exercise risk factors before embarking on a program. You can be at risk if you:

–        have heart problems
–        often complain of chest pain
–        often feel faint and dizzy
–        have a history of high blood pressure

•        Select activities that you enjoy doing, like swimming or walking.

• Listen to your body. Find a time and place that will be suitable for your personality and condition. If you happen to feel more relaxed, and have less pain and more energy in the evenings, by all means exercise in the evenings, as long as it is at least four hours before bedtime.

• Once you start, please be regular in order to gain most of the rewards of exercise.

• Exercise at your own comfortable pace. Watch out for unusual amounts of pain, breathlessness or dizziness.

• Wear appropriate clothes depending on weather, and comfortable shoes.

• Spice up your exercise program with variety. Find exercise partners who have your level of conditioning. These can support and motivate you.

• Set some goals, small and achievable, and challenge yourself. Reward yourself for your goal achievements.

• It is normal for your pulse to be faster; some minor palpitations, sweating, deeper and faster breathing.

• Abnormal symptoms to watch out for include: Chest pain or heaviness in the chest area, pronounced palpitations and breathlessness, especially for minor exertions; wheezing; nausea and faintness; numbness or too much pain.

• In case of injury during exercise, perform the following first aid:

    –     Protect the injured area from further assault.

    –     Rest the injured area.

    –     Apply a cold compress to reduce swelling if any or stop bleeding.

Resume exercise program as pain and injury permits

How Much Exercise Should You Do?

Like I mentioned earlier on, listen to your body. Exercise intensity is usually a combination of how often, how hard and how long you exercise. Simple rules or guidelines you can follow include:

• Don't continue when there is too much pain.

• Exercise about three times a week; that is, on alternate days.

• How hard? Exercise within your heart-rate zone.

• How long? Usually 20 to 30 minutes at a time.

What to Do About Constant Muscle Soreness and Pain

Muscle soreness or pain is usually due to lack of adequate blood flow and the oxygen and nutrients it carries. It is also due to a build-up of metabolites like lactic acid.

Fibromyalgia patients are advised to take a warm prolonged bath before their exercise and fitness program. A warm bath promotes blood circulation and therefore more oxygen to the muscle tissues, which in turn will help flush out the metabolites.

Perhaps the best exercise program for fibromyalgia and other chronic pain patients is swimming or pool exercise activity, with the pool temperature at about 88°.

What is Your Activity Lifestyle Level?

A turtle or a hare? You have a "turtle" or sedentary lifestyle if you spend most of your time in the following activities:

- Frequent naps
- Too much TV
- Writing
- Sewing or needlework
- In the car, bus or train when you venture out

You could have a "hare's" or moderate activity lifestyle if you spend significant amounts of time doing the following:

- Walking at about four miles an hour
- Raking leaves
- Mopping floors
- Walking up and down stairs

Some benefits of improving your activity lifestyle level include:

- You can significantly reduce your risk of heart disease and stroke.

- Reduce your body fat and avoid the complications of obesity.

- You build and preserve your muscles, and improve your metabolic rate.

- Exercise can break your stress cycle and improve your depressive moods.

- It will improve your self-esteem, confidence and your social life.

- Exercise will improve your endurance and stamina, make you less prone to injury and boost your immune system.

Fibromyalgia Exercise and Fitness Program

This would comprise:

- Breathing Exercise
- Stretching Program
- Aerobic Exercise
- Strength Training

In order for exercise to be beneficial for you, adequate planning is essential. The more frequently you exercise, the less time you will need to achieve results. Try not to overdo things. Your exercise program ought to contain the above four types.

I will encourage you to perform some type of exercise daily. You will soon get used to it and you will love it. This is one addiction that can do you a ton of good. If you choose to exercise daily, a simple plan would be to perform an alternate enjoyable activity between a stretching, aerobic or strength-training day. Please use light weights for strengthening. I am advocating you use gravity, light ankle or wrist weights, and exercise rubber bands used in physical therapy centers.

Limit strength training to not more than three times a week initially. This is because your muscle fibers need some time to recover. On the activity day, you may just walk around the block or in a park.

Warm-Up Session

Warm-up is a necessary pre-condition for a safe exercise program. The reasons for this

include:

•       It will improve your exercise performance by promoting your body's circulatory adjustment, minimizing loss of oxygen and decreasing formation of lactic acid.

•       It increases muscle core temperature, which in turn will improve muscle efficiency and oxygen utilization.

•       It allows a quicker blood flow to your lungs.

•       A warm-up session makes you less prone to exercise injuries.

A warm-up session is usually 10 minutes of stretching exercises; whole body gradual movements like in calisthenics; yoga or running very slowly. Keep your heart rate at about 20 beats per minute.

Cool-Down Session

Just like you need a warm-up session before exercise, you will also need a cool-down session. Good reasons for this include:

•       It will prevent the pooling of blood in the extremities.

•       It prevents fainting by increasing blood flow to your heart and brain.

•       It helps prevent cardiac complications like arrhythmias.

A cool-down session is basically the same as a warm-up session. Perform some stretching or calisthenics for approximately 5 to 8 minutes after your exercise program.

Stretching Program

Stretching is a general term used to describe a purposeful maneuver designed to elongate pathologically shortened soft tissues like muscles, thereby increasing the range of movement.

Flexibility is similar to and often used interchangeably with stretching. It is the ability of a soft tissue, like a muscle, to relax and yield to a stretching force.

Our sample stretching program will include the following groups of exercise:

1.   Group A: Hip, Trunk Rotation, Hamstring and Piriformis Muscle Stretch Program. Please study figures 15-1 to 15-9.

2.   Group B: Neck Stretching Program. Please study Figures 15-10a & b; 15-11a & b; 15-12a, b & c ; 15-13 a & b; 15-14a, b & c; 15-15a & b.

3.     Group C: Therapy Ball Stretching Program:

a.     Trunk Side Stretch (figure 15-16)

b.     Shoulder and Torso Stretch (figure 15-17)

c.     Pelvic Tilting Exercise (Abdominal & Back Stretch) (figures 15-18a, b, c & d)

d.     Pelvic Circles Stretch (figure 15-19)

e.     Inner Thigh Stretch (figure 15-20)

f.     Piriformis Stretch (figure 15-21)

g.　Calf and Hamstring Stretch (figure 15-22)

h.　Side to Side Hip Stretch (figure 15-23a, b & c)

i.　Relaxation Bounce (figure 15-24)

4.　Group D: Spinal Mobilization Using a Foam Roller (figures 15-25a, b & c)

5.　TMJ (Temporo-mandibular Joint) Exercise Program (figure 15-26)

## GROUP A: HIP, TRUNK ROTATION, HAMSTRING AND PIRIFORMIS MUSCLE STRETCH PROGRAM

*Group A: Hip, Trunk Rotation, Hamstring and Piriformis Muscle Stretch Program*

**Figure 15-1: Pelvic Tilt**
Place a rolled-up towel underneath your waist; press down on it while contracting your abdominal muscles and tilting your pelvis backward; hold for 5 to 10 seconds.

**Figure 15-2: Knee to Chest**
Bring each knee individually up to chest, pull and hold for 5-10 seconds; alternate.

**Figure 15-3: Both Knees to Chest**
Repeat as in figure 15-2, but bring both knees to chest at the same time.

**Figure 15-4: Trunk Rotation**
Bend and keep knees together as shown, keeping feet on the floor. Stabilize upper trunk and rotate side to side. Hold for 5 to 10 seconds at the end of the rotation to each side.

**Figure 15-5: Hamstring Stretch**
Straighten your knee and stretch with both hands on the calf and hold for 5 to 10 seconds. You can also place your heel against the wall and move your buttocks towards it. (Two-joint muscles like the hamstring easily get shortened with inactivity.)

3. Group C: Therapy Ball Stretching Program:
   a.        Trunk Side Stretch (figure 15-16)

**Figure 15-6: Prayer Stretch**
Feel your back, shoulders and ankles stretch. Hold for 5 to 10 seconds.

**Figure 15-7: Hip Flexor Muscles Stretch**
Assume position and stretch the muscles in front of your hips. Do both limbs. Hold for 5 to 10 seconds.

**Figure 15-8:**
**Hip Abduction**
Bend both knees, as in illustration. Keeping one limb steady, move the other completely away. Alternate between both limbs.

**Figure 15-9: Piriformis Stretch**
Bend and internally rotate your hip with both hands as shown. Hold for 5 to 10 seconds and release.

*Group B: Neck Stretching Program.*
*Repeat Each Exercise Five Times.*

**Figures 15-10a & b: Chin to Chest**
Stand or sit in front of a mirror. While maintaining a good posture, slowly bring your chin toward your chest. Hold for 5 to 10 seconds and return to starting position.

**Figures 15-11a, b & c: Ear to Shoulder**
Tilt your head toward right first, and then the left, as if to touch the shoulder with your ear. Hold each side for 5 to 10 seconds.

**Figures 15-12a & b: Head to Back**

While maintaining position of figure 15-11, move head backward. Keep your upper trunk steady and move only at the neck as you look at the ceiling. Hhold for 5 to 10 seconds and return.

**Figures 15-13a, b & c: Side Turns**

While maintaining position of figure 15-12, gently turn your head to the right or left to look over your shoulder. Hold for 5 to 10 seconds and return.

**Figures 15-14a & b: Oblique Neck Muscles Stretch**
Start as in position in figure 15-14a, grasp your chair for support, and grasp the back of your head with the opposite hand. Turn your head and look at the thigh opposite the hand holding onto the chair. Stretch and hold for 5 to 10 seconds. Alternate.

Figure 15-5: Hamstring Stretch

Straighten your knee and stretch with both hands on the calf and hold for 5 to 10 seconds. You can also place your heel against the wall and move your buttocks towards it. (Two joint muscles like the hamstring easily get shortened with inactivity.)

GROUP B: NECK STRETCHING PROGRAM. REPEAT EACH EXERCISE 5 TIMES.

Figures 15-10a & b: Chin to Chest

Stand or sit in front of a mirror. While maintaining a good posture, slowly bring your chin towards your chest. Hold for 5-10 seconds and return to starting position.

Figures 15-11a, b & c: Ear to Shoulder

Tilt your head towards right and left as if to touch shoulder with ear. Hold for 5-10 seconds.

Figures 15-12a & b: Head to Back

While maintaining previous position, move head backwards. Keep your upper trunk steady and move only at the neck as you look at the ceiling. Hold for 5-10 seconds and return.

Figures 15-13a, b & c: Side Turns

While maintaining previous position, gently turn your head towards the right or left to look over your shoulder. Hold for 5-10 seconds and return.

Figures 15-14a & b: Oblique Neck Muscles Stretch

Start as in previous exercises, grasp your sitting base for support, and grasp the back of your heel with the opposite hand. Turn your head and look at thigh opposite to hand. Stretch and hold for 5-10 seconds. Alternate.

GROUP C: THERAPY BALL STRETCHING PROGRAM
Equipment needed: Therapy or exercise ball of appropriate inflation and size.

| Ball Size | Body Height |
|---|---|
| 45 cm | 55" to 60" |
| 55 cm | 61" to 66" |
| 65 cm | 67" to 71" |
| 75 cm | 72" to 75" |
| 85 cm | 75"+ |

Source of information: Thera-Bond™ Hygenic Corporation
Benefits of Ball Exercises

According to Caroline Corning Creager, a well-known therapy expert, therapy ball exercises have many benefits "too numerous to list." According to her, some of these include:

- Muscle tension relaxation
- Easily provides a total body stretching program
- Improves muscle blood flow
- Assists in body-awareness development
- Assists with positive correction and spine alignment

• Helps relieve depressive moods while energizing the body

• It is fun and entertaining for everyone in the family.

This is a low-impact exercise activity that I highly recommend to fibromyalgia sufferers. The effort at balancing on the ball elicits and exercises all postural muscles. Endurance and strength are also developed as your muscles contract in an eccentric manner. In eccentric contraction, your muscles lengthen as they develop tension and contract to control movement produced by an external force. The therapy ball program involves the following substrates:

1. Trunk Side Stretch
2. Torso Rotational Stretch
3. Abdominal and Back Muscles Stretch (Pelvic Tilt)
4. Pelvic Circles Stretch
5. Inner Thigh Stretch
6. Piriformis Stretch
7. Calf and Hamstring Stretch
8. Side to Side Hip Stretch
9. Relaxation Bounce

**Figure 15-15:**
**Trunk Side Stretch**
　　Keep hip steady with one hand. Raise the opposite arm overhead while bending at the waist until the side is fully stretched. Hold for 5 to 10 seconds. Repeat for the other side.

**Figure 15-16:**
**Torso Rotational Stretch**
　　Sit steady on the ball. With arms raised and extended and hips steady, rotate torso fully towards the left. Hold for 5 to 10 seconds. Repeat to the right. Note that head and upper body should move in unison.

Figure 15-15: Trunk Side Stretch

Keep hip steady with one hand. Raise the opposite arm overhead while bending at the waist until the side is fully stretched. Hold for 5-10 seconds. Repeat for the other side.

Figure 15-16: Torso Rotational Stretch

Sit steady on the ball. With arms raised and extended, and hips steady, rotate torso fully towards the left and the right. Hold for 5-10 seconds. Note that head and upper body should move in unison.

**Figures 15-17a, b & c:
Abdominal/Back Muscles
Stretch (Pelvic Tilt)**

Tilt your pelvis anteriorly
and posteriorly with the
abdominal and back muscles
establishing your movement
axis at the hips while rolling
the ball forward and backward. Perform 10 times.

Figures 15-17a, b & c: Abdominal/Back Muscles Stretch (Pelvic Tilt)

Tilt your pelvis anteriorly and posteriorly with the abdominal and back muscles with movement axis at the hips while rolling ball forwards and backwards.

**Figure 15-18:**
**Pelvic Circles Stretch**
Keeping upper body steady, make circular motions with your hips on the ball. Increase circle size as tolerated. Perform 10 times.

Figure 15-18: Pelvic Circles Stretch

Keeping upper body steady, make circular motions with your hips on the ball. Increase circle size as tolerated.

**Figure 15-19:**
**Inner Thigh Stretch**
Sit steadily on ball as shown. Place both hands on the hips and move legs behind the ball as inner thigh is stretched. Hold for 5 to 10 seconds.

Figure 15-19: Inner Thigh Stretch

Sit steadily on ball as shown. Place both hands on the hips, move legs behind ball as inner thigh is stretched. Hold for 5-10 seconds.

**Figure 15-20:**
**Piriformis Stretch**

Maintain your sitting balance on the ball as shown. Keep your right hand on the ball as you bend your left knee and place the ankle on your right knee. With your left hand on your left knee, gently press down and feel the stretch as your hip rotates internally. Repeat same procedure for the other limb. Hold for 5 to 10 seconds.

Figure 15-20: The Piriformis Stretch

Maintain your sitting balance on ball as shown. Keep your right hand on the ball as you bend left knee and place ankle on right knee. With your left hand on left knee, gently press down and feel the stretch as hip rotates internally. Repeat same procedure for the other limb.

**Figure 15-21: Calf/Hamstring Stretch**
Keep steady on the ball as shown. With both hands firmly planted on left knee, lean forward from the waist. Stretch right knee. Hold for 5 to 10 seconds. Repeat with the other leg.

Figure 15-21: Calf/Hamstring Stretch

Keep steady on the ball as shown. With both hands firmly planted on left knee, lean forward from the waist. Stretch right knee. Hold for 5-10 seconds. Repeat with the other leg.

**Figures 15-22a, b & c:
Side to Side Hip Stretch**
Sit steadily on the ball.
While keeping your upper
torso steady, sway hips from
side to side as shown. Perform
motion 10 times.

Figure 15-22a, b & c: Side to Side Hip Stretch

Sit steadily on the ball. While keeping your upper torso steady, sway hips from side to side as shown.

**Figure 15-23: Relaxation Bounce**
Sit on ball with knees apart. Bounce up and down, with your arms hanging loosely by your sides. Feel gravity pull at your shoulders. The jaw and spine also relax. Perform 10 to 15 times.

Figure 15-23: Relaxation Bounce

Sit on ball with knees apart. Bounce up and down, with your arms hanging loosely by your sides. Feel gravity pull at your shoulders. The jaw and spine also relax.

## GROUP D: SPINAL MOBILIZATION USING AN EXERCISE FOAM ROLLER

The spinal column is made up of several postural muscles and ligaments that originate and attach in oblique directions on the articulating facets. These maintain the normal "S" shaped curvature of the spine. The flexibility of the curves enables the spine to withstand 10 times more axial compression forces than if it were a straight column instead. Balance and flexibility in the spinal system is necessary to counteract the effects of gravity and other external forces.

By rolling up and down and side to side, the tiny joints and muscles of the spine can be stretched.

**Figure 15-24a**
While lying down on the foam roller, parallel with it, slowly roll from side to side. Extend one arm. Perform this 10 times.

**Figure 15-24b**
While maintaining position in figure 15-24a, slowly raise both arms up and down. Perform 10 times.

**Figure 15-24c**
Lie down on the roller, perpendicular to it. Cushion head with both arms. Gently and slowly roll up and down your spine. Perform 10 times.

Figure 15-24a

While lying down parallel on the foam roller, slowly roll from side to side. Extend one arm. Perform this 10 times.

Figure 15-24b

While maintaining position 15-24a, slowly raise both arms up and down. Perform about 10 times.

Figure 15-24c

Lie down perpendicular on the roller. Cushion head with both arms. Gently and slowly roll up and down your spine. Repeat 10 times.

**Figure 15-25: Temporomandibular Joint Exercise**
Place two fingers together on the side of your jaw.
Try to resist your jaw movements with the fingers.

TMJ Exercise Program

Many fibromyalgia patients have problems with their temporo-mandibular joints. Muscles would get tight quite easily if not used often and create a lot of pain which often radiates to this area of the face.

Some TMJ Problem Tips

• Cut up your food into tiny bits, so you don't have to open your mouth too widely.

• Eat very soft foods, avoid tough meat, etc.

• Avoid chewing gum.

• Don't form a habit of biting off food with front teeth.

• If you clench and grind teeth at night, you might consider asking your dentist for an appropriate prosthesis or bite pads.

Method

Place two fingers together on the side of your jaw. Try to resist your jaw movements with the fingers.

Aerobic Exercise and Fibromyalgia

Several studies attest to the fact that aerobic and cardio-vascular fitness activities are superior and more effective than any other type of exercise program in treating fibromyalgia symptoms.

As I mentioned at the beginning of this chapter, exercise, especially aerobic, should be built up gradually. The eventual aim is to exercise for 20 to 30 minutes at a target heart rate of 60% to 80% of your maximum heart rate.

Exercise Basics

Fitness

This is a general term which has different meanings to different people, depending on their sex, age, heredity, activity level and disease condition. For the fibromyalgia or chronic pain patient, it is the ability to perform activities of daily living without feelings of exertion or fatigue. Fitness depends on endurance.

Endurance

This is the ability to perform work for a prolonged period of time, while resisting fatigue. It depends on your body's level of oxygen utilization. The amount of oxygen your body gets in a minute would eventually depend on your cardiovascular fitness. This can be greatly enhanced by exercising at your target heart rate for a prolonged amount of time.

Aerobic Exercise

This is the next step above a moderate-intensity activity. It is simply an extended activity that makes you breathe harder, and your heart beat faster. The best aerobic exercise is any activity you enjoy and can perform for about 20 minutes at your target heart zone.

Examples include:
- Brisk walking
- Jogging
- Bicycling
- Stair climbing
- Aerobic dance
- Skiing

Target Heart Rate

Your maximum heart rate is determined by subtracting your age from 220. Your target heart rate is the rate you achieve through exercise to a zone between 60% to 80% of your maximum heart rate. For example, if you are 40 years old, your maximum heart rate is 180 (220 – 40). You should exercise and aim for 108 to 144 beats per minute (60% to 80% of 180).

Target Heart Rate By Age

| AGE | 60% | 80% |
|-----|-----|-----|
| 30 | 114 | 152 |
| 35 | 111 | 148 |
| 40 | 108 | 144 |
| 45 | 105 | 140 |
| | | |

| | | |
|-----|-----|-----|
| 50 | 102 | 136 |
| 55 | 99 | 132 |
| 60 | 96 | 128 |
| 65 | 93 | 124 |

How to Measure Heart Rate

Exercise for a while. Stop and place first two fingers (not thumb) on the base of thumb in front of the wrist of opposite hand. Locate a pulse. Watch the second indicator of your watch. Count your pulse for 15 seconds, then multiply this count by 4 to get your heart rate.

High-Impact Aerobics

Aerobics in which both feet come off the ground in different choreography styles.

Low-Impact Aerobics (Recommended for Fibromyalgia Patients)

Aerobic exercise in which one foot is always planted firmly on the ground.

Body-Sculpting Aerobics

Aerobic exercise combined with free weight exercise program, aimed at toning the body and improving muscular strength.

Funk Aerobics

A combination of low- and high-impact dance movements. It can be rock, or cardio-funk.

Muscle-Strengthening Exercise (Progressive Resistance Exercise)

This is defined as any form of exercise or activity in which muscle action (whether static or dynamic) is opposed by an outside force. Muscles gain strength, endurance, and power when they habitually work against an opposite force like gravity, free weights, ankle weights, etc.

You need muscle-strengthening activity in order to develop endurance or fight fatigue during performance of activities of daily living.

This statement usually conjures up images of weird-looking muscle builders, and several hours at the gym every day. The fact of the matter is that you don't need anything more than mild strengthening to tone your body and build endurance. However, you need to be regular at it.

## SAMPLE MUSCLE-STRENGTHENING PROGRAM

A. To strengthen extensor group of muscles of the wrist, arms, neck, back and hips.

**Figures 15-26a, b, c, & d**
Graded in increasing degrees of resistance (Progressive Resistance) starting with just the weight of your arms, legs and gravity. Hold each position for 5 to 10 seconds.

Figure 15-26a, b, c, and d. Graded in increasing degrees of resistance (Progressive Resistance) starting with just the weight of your arms, legs and gravity.

B. To strengthen the flexor group of muscles – (abdominal muscles, hip muscles, thighs).

**Figures 15-27a, b, & c.**
Lie on the floor or a bed. Gradually increase resistance as shown.

Lie on the floor or bed as in Figures 15-27a, b, & c. Gradually increase resistance as shown.

**Figure 15-28**

Use cuff weights strapped around your ankles and wrists or work out with dumbbells as shown.

A. Grasp a dumbbell in each hand as shown. Raise the dumbbells to shoulder height. From this starting position, raise the dumbbells above your head until your elbows are fully extended. Repeat 10 to 20 times (as tolerated.

B. Strap a lightweight weight cuff around each ankle. Raise legs alternately until knees are fully extended. Hold for 5 to 10 seconds. Repeat 10 times.

## How to Benefit Fully From Your Exercise And Fitness Program

Set Sensible Goals

Stay motivated by reminding yourself often about the benefits you hope to achieve if you persevere in your program. Actually write them down and read them often. Set sensible, achievable short-term goals, like being able to mop your kitchen floor without fatigue.

• Maintain an Exercise Journal. Write down symptoms and problems encountered. You may need to discuss this with your doctor, trainer or physical therapist.

• Reward yourself each time you are able to achieve a goal.

A good motivation for hanging in there is the thought of the immense relief you will get from depressive moods, pain, fatigue, and improvement in your sleep quality. The list is endless. Most importantly, this is the only way I know you can completely take back your life from fibromyalgia.

Tips on How to Maintain a Fitness-Conscious Lifestyle

• Create situations what will make you exercise, like parking your car far away, so you get to walk the distance.

• Spend time with the kids outdoors if the weather permits.

• Get an exercise partner of the same fitness level and take long walks.

• Use the stairs instead of the elevator whenever you can.

• Include some form of exercise activity in your daily activity planner.

A SAMPLE PROGRAM CAN BE:

• 20 min. stretching and aerobics 3x/week.

• Strengthening and activity (walking) 2x/week.

At the least, endeavor to include 20 minutes of aerobics 2 times a week. Stretching can be done any time you can.

# Chapter 16: Fast Solutions For Muscle Soreness, Headaches and Sleep Problems

## A. MUSCLE SORENESS

1. A good night's sleep: Getting a good night's sleep may be the solution for most muscle soreness problems. In fibromyalgia, for example, muscle soreness can be traced to lack of restorative sleep. As discussed earlier on in this book, the deep phase of sleep is required for the repairing hormone from the pituitary gland to become effective in repairing muscle micro-trauma. Therefore, forming a good sleep hygiene habit would go a long way to alleviating this problem.

2. Mind your posture: The postural muscles of your body are in constant tension, both static and dynamic, in maintaining your erect body in space against the pull of gravity. These muscles function optimally when your body is balanced over its center of gravity. In this situation, muscles in all sides of the body are in equilibrium, and contract efficiently. If you stoop, for example, and move beyond this line of gravity, muscles in the back will contract to prevent you from falling forward and vice versa.

If a poor posture situation becomes habitual, these opposing muscles sometimes become tired and sore. In order to relieve this fatigue and soreness, you must manage the predisposing factor, which is poor posture.

Good Posture Hints

•Watch out for your head position. Correct it and the rest of the body will follow. Gently tuck in your chin as you stretch the muscles at the back of the neck.

•Brace and pull your shoulders backwards.

•Practice often at aligning your ear, shoulder, hips and ankle. Visualize an invisible line that passes through these four structures, and your task is to maintain it in a straight line.

•Always remember to sit straight, while maintaining the natural curve inwards of your lower back. Also make sure your car's seat is ergonomically designed to assist you in maintaining a correct posture. If not, buy a posture correction insert.

•Sleep on a mattress that is firm enough not to sag under your weight, and soft enough to adapt to the natural curves of your body. If you suffer from back pain, you might consider sleeping in a "neutral" or "zero gravity" position (See figure 14-3 in Chapter 14).

•Change positions often; that is, don't stand or sit for more than 20 minutes at a time.

•Shoes: Avoid high-heeled shoes, platform shoes, high boots and others with inflexible soles. Keep your shoe heel height at about 1.8" to 2.5" and don't wear them for too long.

•Bags and weights: Avoid heavy luggage, ask someone to help you. Don't strap over shoulders. Keep close to the body. If you have to lift, bend at the knees, instead of the waist.

•Bras: Heavy breasts tend to pull a woman forward, and promote a rounded shoulder posture. Wear a strong bra that crosses over at the back. Don't let them fit too tightly around the chest or over the shoulders, because this can restrict blood flow or put pressure on spinal nerves.

3. Warm baths: Soak yourself in a warm aromatic bath for about an hour. Set a timer in case you fall asleep and hurt yourself. You can also light an aromatic candle and listen to relaxation music.

4. Over-the-counter medication: Try these first before using addictive prescription painkillers. Be on a SAM e supplementation program. Medical research has proven that SAM e can relieve muscle pain even better than a TENS unit.

5. TENS units: This is a kind of electrical stimulator used in most physical therapy centers. You may have to order through a physical therapist or your physician.

6. Trigger point injections: An anti-inflammatory steroid can be injected directly into the painful site. I am not sure how helpful this can be for fibromyalgia pain which essentially is different from inflammatory symptoms.

7. Breathing/muscle relaxation exercise: Breathing exercises have a general calming effect on your system. More oxygen eventually gets to your muscles. Minor muscle spasms may have created muscle tension and pain. Twenty minutes of deep muscle relaxation exercise (see Chapter 14) can perform miracles on your pain.

B.   HEADACHES

It is very important that you are thoroughly evaluated for the cause or causes of your regular headaches. Find a physician who has some experience with headaches and has a kind of headache program or clinic.

If you experience nausea, drowsiness, vomiting and fever, you really need to be evaluated by a doctor. Causes of headaches can range from mild spasms of the head and neck muscles to very serious disease conditions.

Standard painkillers usually relieve regular headaches. There are medications that resolve blood vessel changes, etc.

Some self-help strategies include:

• Stress and muscle tension management (Chapter 14)

• Check for allergies and sensitivity to particular substances or foods.

• Get plenty of fresh air, enough sleep and rest.

• Avoid caffeine and any other foods that have been known to trigger off your headaches. Keep a headache diary.

• Check your pillow and neck posture while sleeping. Get appropriate neck support or pillow.

• Get a deep massage. You can also use a massager. Some come with a heat and vibration control.

• Aromatherapy: Lavender essential oil mixed with almond oil can be used to massage head and neck muscles. Other oils commonly used include peppermint and eucalyptus.

• Breathing Exercises: Chronic headaches result in fatiguing of head and neck muscles, due to constant tension. This reduces muscle blood flow as blood vessels are contracted. Less oxygen gets to the muscles and lactic acid builds up. This causes more pain and tension as the vicious cycle continues. Deep diaphragmatic breathing and rest can break up this cycle.

Sleep Problems

Lack of sleep, otherwise called insomnia, is a common human problem that affects about 10% to 15% of the population, mostly women. There are several types of insomnia, and the problem can include:

- Problem with initiating sleep
- Problem with remaining asleep
- Circadian rhythm problems
- Restless legs and other uncontrollable muscle activity associated with sleep
- And of course lack of deep phase of sleep, leading to unrestorative sleep

In order to accurately diagnose the problem, a medical expert needs to conduct a thorough evaluation. It may be necessary to be tested in a sleep laboratory. Many prescription sleep medications are very addictive. This can happen in as little as one week of medication.

In minor cases of insomnia, the problem can be resolved with regular relaxation training and deep breathing exercises. Sleep as a biological process should not be controlled or made to happen, it should rather be allowed to happen by observing some simple sleep hygiene:

- Avoid caffeine, alcohol, nicotine and other chemical stimulants.
- Don't watch television, especially intense programs, just before bedtime.
- Put a leash on your mind, avoid worrying during bedtime, limit your worrying to a designated "worry time."
- Get plenty of exercise or aerobic activity during the day. Don't exercise, however, too close to your bedtime. Give at least a four-hour gap.

• Take a walk in the early morning sunshine. This may help reset your body's internal clock.

• Practice prayer and meditation.

• Avoid prolonged naps during the day. This will impair quality of your sleep later in the day.

• Let the bedroom be a good place to sleep. Avoid turning it into something else, like another office.

• Create a pre-sleep program or ritual, like read a passage from a helpful book, listen to soft music, etc.

• Eat lightly before bedtime. Too much food, close to your bedtime, is enough to prevent you from falling asleep.

• Endeavor to maintain a regular bedtime and waking time.

• Improve on your bedroom environment with soft sleep aids, pillows and assistive devices that can assist you in relaxing.

• Maintain a neutral or zero gravity sleeping posture. This will reduce muscle tension significantly.

• If you think you have sleep apnea, please get a medical check-up to correct the problem.

• Take a long warm bath or steam bath before sleep time.

• I personally find relaxation sound tapes (waterfalls, rains, forest sounds) very relaxing.

# Chapter 17: Nutritional Healing

The quality of our lives is very much affected by what we eat or inhale that a very large part of what we know as alternative medicine has been built on the manipulation of what we eat and drink.

Our bodies require all sorts of nutrients to survive – for energy, growth and tissue repair. Most of our bodies are composed of water, which acts as a medium for blood and plasma, transporting nutrients into tissue cells and evacuating their waste products.

Macronutrients comprise protein, fats and carbohydrates; proteins are required for tissue growth and maintenance and the formation of several hormones and enzymes; fat, on the other hand, provides energy, insulates organs, and assists with the utilization of certain vitamins. Carbohydrates are the body's chief energy reservoir.

Micronutrients include vitamins and minerals. These nutrients, even though needed in small amounts, are vital to the body's health. Prolonged deficiency can cause numerous health problems.

Other Methylation Boosters

Many people complain about the exorbitant cost of SAM e. In fact, regular supplementation with SAM e can cost upward of $200 per month. As an alternative, it is important to note that other nutrients are quite capable of boosting methylation.

Folic Acid, Vitamin B6, (Pyridoxal S-phosphate) and Vitamin B12 (Cobalamin)

These play a major role in assisting the body to achieve an optimal utilization of SAM e. They also play a major role in the breakdown of a harmful amino acid called homocysteine.

Homocysteine can be beneficial in small amounts, since it is associated with transsulfuration and methylation reactions. The homocysteine molecule contains highly useful sulfur substrates. Excessive amounts, however, can lead to serious liver and heart problems.

Homocysteine levels in the body are controlled through enzymatic degradation. This process requires adequate levels of folate and vitamins B6 and B13 to maintain a normal balance between homocysteine and SAM e. Or, as you take SAM e, you might want to includes a 'B' complex multivitamin.

According to recent medical research, you will need about 650 micrograms of folic acid daily in order to significantly lower homocysteine levels in your system. A British study, using a large number of participants, reported a dramatic reduction in their homocysteine levels with a dosage of 500 micrograms of folic acid.

How to Use B6, B12 and Folic Acid

These are produced in different varieties and shapes, tablets and capsules, either singly or as B-complex preparations. An effective dosage is 500 to 750 micrograms of folic acid.

According to Ms. Corinne Netzer's Big Book of Medical Cures, it is better to take all three, since they cooperate and influence each other.

Are There Any Side Effects?

Of course, as they say that too much of a good thing is bad. Very high doses of the 'B' vitamins may cause gas, bloating, gastric upsets and diarrhea. Also long-term usage can cause kidney problems. So check with your doctor if you are taking more than 800 micrograms of folic acid daily.

## Fibromyalgia Symptoms and Supplements

Many alternative health practitioners believe strongly that the key to fibromyalgia care is well-planned nutrition and supplementation. Besides SAM e, several other nutrients have been found helpful for the following diseases:

- Muscle soreness
- Sleep problems
- Chronic fatigue
- Cognitive impairment, also called fibro-fog
- Headaches and migraines
- Irritable bowel syndrome

## Muscle Soreness

Several theories have been postulated about the cause of muscle soreness in fibromyalgia. Most of them point to a lack of restorative sleep as the culprit. Muscle soreness is normally remedied during the deep phase of sleep, also known as Stage 4, by the action of a hormone secreted by the pituitary gland. Another theory implicates a local lack of oxygen by muscle tissues, leading to a decrease of glycogen breakdown and the synthesis of ATP. Because of the aforementioned theories, many experts believe adequate supplementation with malic acid and magnesium would resolve muscle pain or soreness.

Malic Acid and Magnesium

We normally get malic acid into our bodies throughout diet. It can also be produced in small quantities by our bodies during the citric acid cycle. Malic acid is very important for energy production during both aerobic and anaerobic processes. Actually, a research study was undertaken to determine its effects under diminished muscle oxygen states (like in fibromyalgia). The researchers noticed significant improvement within 48 hours at a dosage of 1200 to 2400 mg of malic acid.

### How to Take Malic Acid

It comes in tablets of 250 mg each. Take 500 to 750 mg of malic acid about 1 hour before breakfast and another 500 mg before dinner.

Magnesium

Magnesium is the most important supplement for energy production and mitochondria health. Low levels of magnesium can disrupt ATP production. Because ATP energizes the movement of magnesium into cells, a vicious cycle is set in motion which further hampers ATP synthesis. Several studies seem to suggest that magnesium, when combined with malic acid, reduced tender points by 41% after only four weeks of treatment.

How to Take Magnesium

Magnesium comes in tablet form. It may be combined with other nutrients as a multivitamin. An effective daily does is about 300 to 600 mg, usually taken with regular meals to encourage optimal absorption.

Side Effects: May cause stomach upsets and diarrhea.

Sleep Problems

As discussed already, non-restorative sleep is a primary cause of the symptoms of fibromyalgia. This is a situation where the deep phase of sleep is interrupted by awake-like bursts of brain activity. Recommended supplements include melatonin and valerian root.

Melatonin is produced naturally by the pineal gland. Besides being a powerful anti-oxidant, it greatly affects the body's sleep/awake cycle. It has been found to be a good sleep problem remedy without the side effects associated with sleeping pills.

## How to Take Melatonin

It comes in tablet forms of 2.5 mg each. Take one tablet at bedtime, usually as a small sublingual tablet.

Boosting Your Melatonin Level Naturally

Melatonin has a Dracula-like attitude: Its levels rise with the sunset and continues through the night. Then it starts to decrease with daylight. This in turn triggers off neural impulses which slow melatonin production.

Besides this rhythmic cycle of light and darkness, other factors like daily routine may play some role. Some experts suggest the following melatonin lifestyle may boost its natural production:

• Eat meals regularly. This will ensure a regular body rhythm.

• Eat light meals at night. Digestion process slows down with melatonin production.

• Avoid stimulants like coffee, tea or caffeine-containing medicines.

• Don't exercise too late at night, as this can delay melatonin production. Take a walk outside at sunrise.

Caution With Melatonin

Please be advised that melatonin is a powerful hormone. Any artificial regulation may have profound effects in your body. Dr. Gary Richardson, an assistant professor of medicine at Brown University, believes that supplementation of melatonin can add to your sleep problem. Melatonin falls within an FDA non-regulated area, and so certain dosages may increase melatonin process to abnormal levels.

Valerian Root

Known to have been used by ancient Greeks to cure insomnia. The Europeans use it for anxiety and restlessness, both of which effects can improve sleep quality.

Valerian root is derived from dried rhizomes and plant roots. It contains two distinct substances which affect the central nervous system – vale potriates and sesquiterpenes. They work by slowing down and sedating the central nervous system and the mind.

How to Take Valerian Root

It comes in capsule form of 500 mg valerian root powder per capsule. Take 1 to 3 capsules (about 500-1500 mg), preferably with some food. Valerian root also comes as extracts, tinctures, or in teas.

Side Effects: None. This makes valerian root better as a sleep aid than melatonin.

**Chronic Fatigue**

Recommended supplements for chronic fatigue include NADH, CoEnzyme Q10, malic acid, magnesium and L-carnitine.

NADH (Nicotinamide Adenine Dinucleotide) Also Known as CoEnzyme 1

This is a nutrient that is contained in our diet. It is a nutrient that can enhance the production of dopamine and some other transmitters and also assist in the cells' process of converting food to energy. Dr. Jorg Birkmayer, director of the Birkmayer Institute for Parkinson's Therapy in Vienna, has been using NADH to treat chronic fatigue syndrome patients, among other ailments. He usually prescribed 10 mg of NADH daily before breakfast and has reported significant improvements in health condition within 8 to 12 weeks of treatment.

Another clinician, Dr. Joseph Bellanti of Georgetown University Immunology Center in Washington, DC, found good results in a study involving 26 patients with chronic fatigue syndrome. Nineteen of these reported significant improvements in their condition.

Recommended Dosage: Take 5 to 10 mg. Usually comes in tablet form. There are no known adverse effects and contraindications.

CoEnzyme Q10

This nutrient is produced naturally in the body, and stored in concentrated amounts within the heart muscles. CoEnzyme Q10 is also found in foods, especially organ meats. It is an important nutrient for the body's energy conversion processes like ATP synthesis. It also aids electron transport processes across the mitochondria. Another CoEnzyme Q10 function is to act as a powerful antioxidant within the body.

It is particularly beneficial for heart conditions. It bolsters the heart. It does this by increasing the heart's energy output, making it stronger. Dr. William Lee had called it "the ultimate antidote to aging." Some researchers also believe it may play a role in breast cancer recurrence prevention. CoQ10 also assists in boosting our body's immune response system.

### How to Take CoQ10

Normally packaged in softgels of 100 mg each. Cardiologists usually recommend a dosage of 300 to 300 [CeCe: This is how ms. read; ck w/Dr. E.] mg of CoQ10 daily for heart problems. About 100 mg (one softgel) is recommended for chronic fatigue supplementation.

Malic Acid and Magnesium have already been discussed, in connection with muscle soreness.

L-Carnitine

This is produced in the liver and kidneys. Its function within the body includes fatty acid transfer into cells for energy production. Therefore, regular supplementation with L-carnitine would enhance the processes of fat transport and metabolism. Dr. Plioplys reported significant improvements in 12 out of 18 chronic fatigue patients he had treated with L-carnitine.

This nutrient is known to lower cholesterol levels in the blood; boosts the body against stress; supports kidney, heart and liver functions. It also promotes our body's ability to endure prolonged physical activity.

### How to Take L-Carnitine

Packaged in 250 mg capsules. Take 1 to 3 capsules daily.

Cognitive Impairment (Fibro-Fog)

Cognitive impairment, also called "fibro-fog" among fibromyalgia syndrome sufferers, is a term that describes a gradual short-term memory loss. Patients begin to forget simple things like where they parked their cars or forget all about appointments.

A brain deprived of adequate amounts of oxygen, glucose and other nutrients malfunctions, just like any other organ. Its information processing system becomes impaired.

Probable causes of this in fibromyalgia patients include:

• Insufficient blood supply to the brain

• Stress, which produces excessive amounts of cortisol, which in turn interferes with memory

• Poor nutritional habits

• Medications being used

Probable nutritional remedies include ginkgo biloba, phosphatidyl choline, and acetyl L-carnitine.

Ginkgo Biloba

Ginkgo is known to be the oldest living tree species found on Earth. This tree is believed to contain several antioxidants, like flavonoids like rutin and quercetin, which assist in the degradation of free radicals.

Flavonoids also improve brain blood flow by strengthening capillaries. It prevents the accumulation of brain fluids and activates the brain's chemical messengers.

An ancient Chinese and European remedy was scientifically tested in a major study by LeBars and associations at the New York Institute of Medical Research. About 309 patients with severe memory problems following stroke and Alzheimer's were tested in the study.

After one year of observation, the researchers reported significant improvements in many subjects from the patient group in areas of memory, reasoning, and social functioning than members of the placebo group. They also observed that supplementation with ginkgo biloba was able to arrest the progress of cognitive impairment in some subjects.

How to Take Ginkgo

Packaged in different forms. Best form is capsule form. Take 120 mg daily for memory problems. No side effects have been reported.

Phosphatidyl Choline

This is a major substrate of lecithin. It promotes the emulsification and degradation of fat deposits. Due to this function, phosphatidyl choline is helpful in preventing heart problems; the narrowing of arteries. It also assists in the prevention of liver diseases and gall stones. According to clinical studies, memory impairment can be improved with a 3 g daily dose.

### How to Take Phosphatidyl Choline

Packaged in softgels of 420 mg each. Take about 420 to 840 mg daily (that is, one to two softgels). Pregnant patients should check with their gynecologists. It may be contraindicated.

Acetyl L-Carnitine

This is another naturally occurring substance. Although related to carnitine, it has a different chemical composition. It is another antioxidant and assists in degradation of free radicals. Other functions include promotion of cell health by assisting in cellular energy production.

Dr. Jay Pattegrew of the University of Pittsburgh School of Medicine conducted a clinical study in which 3000 mg of acetyl L-carnitine was used to treat several patients with some form of cognitive impairment for one year. He compared the results from this group against that of the placebo group. He found that the acetyl L-carnitine group performed better on a battery of cognitive status tests than the placebo group. This led Dr. Pattegrew and associates to believe that acetyl L-carnitine may be able to halt memory loss progress in Alzheimer's patients.

### How to Take Acetyl L-Carnitine

Usually packaged in capsules. There are no government dosage guidelines. Clinicians recommend a dosage of 1000 to 3000 mg daily. For best results, take in divided doses throughout the day, on an empty stomach.

Side Effects: No known serious ones. Very few people have reported nausea and vomiting.

### Headaches and Migraines

Causes of headaches and migraines are several and varied. A thorough medical examination by a headache expert and physician is required. This is because the headaches and migraines may be symptoms of a more severe health problem. Also, a comprehensive evaluation is a pre-condition for an effective headache remedy.

Migraine Headache: Pain is caused by changes in blood vessels of the temples. This pain can last for days. Other symptoms of migraine headache include visual problems, nausea and dizziness.

Cluster Headache: Similar to migraine, and also caused by blood vessel changes. Pain is intense and localized around one eye. Pain is intermittent; that is, goes and comes back after a few hours. It is known to last for a long time. Nobody is sure what causes it.

Tension Headache: This type of headache is usually caused by stress and muscle tension, especially tension in the muscles of head and neck. It can also have other causes, like exposure to environmental toxins.

Nutritional remedies for headaches include:

Feverfew

Magnesium

Peppermint oil

Eucalyptus oil

Feverfew

This nutrient has over a two-thousand-year history among herbalists of different cultures. Ancient Greeks used it for painful menstrual periods. It has been used since the 1970s in America and Canada in the prevention or relief of painful headaches. It is especially effective for migraine headaches, but can also effect blood vessels and consequently relieve other headache symptoms.

The first known scientific proof of the effectiveness of feverfew on migraine was conducted by Johnson and associates in 1985 and reported in the British Medical Journal. Seventeen migraine sufferers who had been on a diet of feverfew leaves (which they chewed) were divided into two groups.

One group received feverfew capsules (instead of leaves); the other group got some kind of placebo. On reevaluation after a time, results showed no change in the feverfew group, while the placebo group got worse. Due to this result, the researchers concluded that feverfew was beneficial for headache relief, and it didn't matter whether one took it in capsule form or chewed leaves instead.

## How to Take Feverfew

Packaged in capsule or table forms. It can also be chewed as dried or fresh leaves. There may be some irritation of the mouth for some.

Dosage: Purchase a standardized brand, usually, standardized with 0.2% of parthenolide as an active ingredient. Take a daily does of 250 micrograms of parthenolide or check manufacturer's dosace specification.

Adverse Effects: You may be allergic to it. It may cause rashes or some itching in some people. Pregnant women should be careful and might be better off discussing with their gynecologist. Feverfew can cause uterine contractions.

Magnesium

Research findings indicate some headache sufferers have low levels of magnesium in their systems and supplementation with it has been observed to bring relief from headaches. Mauskop and fellow investigators gave 1000 mg of magnesium intravenously to a mixed group of 40 headache patients which included children, women and men.

The results indicate that headache symptoms were completely eliminated in about 80% of participants in the study. Already, magnesium is known to relieve symptoms like hypersensitivity to light and nausea.

How to Take Magnesium for Headaches

Magnesium comes in tablet form. It can also be combined with other nutrients as a multivitamin preparation. Optimal dosage from several studies is 360 to 600 mg daily, taken at meal time.

Adverse Effects: Usually safe. May cause stomach irritation and diarrhea. Magnesium is contraindicated for people with heart and kidney problems.

### Irritable Bowel Syndrome

Formerly known as spastic colon or mucous colitis. Symptoms include cramps, bloating, gas and changes in bowel habits. Some IBS patients have constipation or diarrhea or both. The medical textbooks say there is no cure. I say perhaps there is, only one hasn't been found yet. Some have also called it a functional disorder and not really a disease, since the colon shows no sign of a disease on examination. But whatever the medical community chooses to call it would not trivialize the serious problems sufferers face continually.

### Nutritional Remedies for IBS

A proper and well-planned diet may relieve symptoms. If you are a sufferer, it is a good idea to maintain a journal of what helps it get better and the things that make it worse, and discuss these with your physician.

A dietician can be consulted to assist you in planning an adequate diet, but do not sacrifice your normal nutritional balance just because you are worried about IBS symptoms. That is, "don't cut off your nose to spite your face." Dietary fiber may help. Whole grain breads, cereals, fruits, beans and vegetables are excellent sources of fiber.

High-fiber diets relieve IBS by mildly distending the colon, thereby preventing intestinal spasms from developing. Fibers also can retain water in stools, thereby making them easier to evacuate.

Peppermint Oil

This substance contains a large quantity of menthol, which is an ancient remedy for intestinal problems. Menthol appears to slow down cramping muscle spasms and also relieves indigestion and diarrhea.

How to Take Peppermint Oil

It is packaged in gelatin or coated capsules. Gelatin packaging is preferred since it will disintegrate easily once in the stomach environment.

For IBS take an enteric-coated capsule. This will allow it to bypass the stomach and break up within the colon, where its action is needed.

For dosage guidelines, please observe the manufacturer's specifications.

There are no known adverse effects.

Psyllium

Also called plantago and ispaghula. Psyllium is primarily used as a laxative and to treat diarrhea. One study involving 26 IBS patients reported some relief of irritable bowel syndrome symptoms in about 20 of the participants in the study.

Dosage: Follow manufacturer's guidelines.

**Good Health Starts With A Good Diet**

THE FOOD GUIDE PYRAMID

The main objective of diet plans is to achieve and maintain an adequate body composition, which will provide an adequate capacity for physical and mental work. The daily requirement of essential nutrients depends on several variables like sex, age, height, weight, metabolic and activity level.

In order to determine an adequate nutritional variation for Americans, the Food and Nutrition Board of the National Academy of Sciences – National Research Council and the US Department of Agriculture analyzed information and data on 45 essential nutrients in people on special diets and came up with the following Food Guide Pyramid.

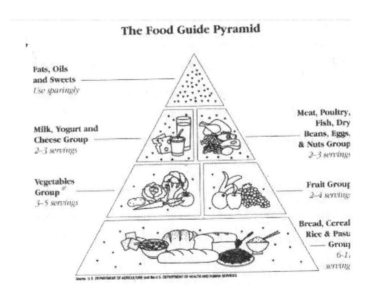

((FDA food pyramid to be inserted))

**What Counts as a Serving?\***

Grain Products Group (bread, cereal, rice, and pasta)
- One slice of bread
- 1 ounce of ready-to-eat cereal
- ½ cup of cooked cereal, rice, or pasta

Vegetable Group
- 1 cup of raw leafy vegetables
- ½ cup of other vegetables – cooked or chopped raw
- ¾ cup of vegetable juice

Fruit Group
- 1 medium apple, banana, orange
- ½ cup of chopped, cooked, or canned fruit
- ¾ cup of fruit juice

Milk Group (milk, yogurt, and cheese)
- 1 cup of milk or yogurt
- 1½ ounces of natural cheese
- 2 ounces of processed cheese

Meat and Beans Group (meat, poultry, fish, dry beans, eggs, and nuts)
- 2-3 ounces of cooked lean meat, poultry, or fish
- ½ cup of cooked dry beans or 1 egg counts as 1 ounce of lean meat. Two tablespoons of peanut butter or 1/3 cup of nuts count as 1 ounce of meat.

\*Some foods fit into more than one group. Dry beans, peas, and lentils can be counted as servings in either the meat and beans group or the vegetable group. These "cross-over" foods can be counted as servings from either one or the other group, but not both. Serving sizes indicated here are those used in the Food Guide Pyramid and based on both suggested and usually consumed portions necessary to achieve adequate nutrient intake. They differ from serving sizes on the Nutrition Facts Label, which reflects portions usually consumed.

In summary, the pyramid offers the following usual advice to Americans:

• Choose a diet with plenty of grain products, vegetables and fruits.

• Choose a diet that is low in fat, saturated fat and cholesterol.

• Eat a variety of foods.

• Choose a diet that is moderate in salt and sodium.

• Choose a diet that is moderate in sugars.

• If you drink alcoholic beverages, please do so in moderation.

Above all, balance what you consume with adequate physical activity, or else you will be climbing a mountain you'll have a tough time coming down from. There are usually no safe fixes or some medications that can make the fat go away. If you put it on, be prepared to take it off with exercise and correction of poor nutritional habits.

# Chapter 18: Fibromyalgia Disability Issues And How To File Claims Successfully

**HOW TO FILE CLAIMS SUCCESSFULLY**.

Why the Social Security Administration (SSA) Routinely Denies Fibromyalgia Disability Claims Applications

One major reason for this is that fibromyalgia sufferers have a hard time proving that they are disabled per SSA criteria. Other reasons include:

• Lack of current work capacity documentation in medical records.

• Lack of objective and quantifiable laboratory findings.

• Constant fatigue and poor endurance are not enough disability indicators.

• Many physicians fail to document clear evidence of disability.

The Social Security Administration is known to routinely deny fibromyalgia-related disability applications except where there are other disabling diagnoses with supporting laboratory data. This is not the case in countries like Canada and many European countries, where fibromyalgia is regarded as a disabling condition.

Therefore, in order to file claims successfully you, your lawyer and physician must function like a team in providing needed medical information, especially evidence of total disability.

This means you cannot function in a recent job and cannot be retrained for any other alternative jobs. The physician's notes are crucial to a successful outcome but unfortunately, many patients often change doctors midstream. Most sufferers understandably differ in opinion as to their healthcare strategies and priorities. And so, there may be cases of patients' non-compliance to their doctors' prescriptions, etc.

Available research data seem to suggest that about 30% of fibromyalgia sufferers change jobs because of their condition. Seventeen percent of them can no longer perform in their previous jobs.

A research study by Wolfe and associates indicates that about 26% of fibromyalgia patients reported receiving one form of disability payment or another. This number increased to 46.4% after 1988. A look at the national trend revealed that the San Antonio and Los Angeles areas had the highest records of disability claims applications.

**The Fibromyalgia Impact Questionnaire (FIQ)**

A very good solution to the perennial problem of lack of disability documentation in fibromyalgia disability insurance claims is the Fibromyalgia Impact Questionnaire (FIQ). See table 18-1.

The FIQ in its original form is a 10-item self-administered questionnaire that can objectively document depression, functional capacity, work capacity, anxiety, sleep, pain, stiffness, fatigue and general well-being. The Fibromyalgia Impact Questionnaire is actually an adaptation from a commonly used arthritis impact questionnaire.

The FIQ is considered an effective tool due to the following reasons:

• Very practical and only needs a short time to complete.

• Its comprehensive nature takes fibromyalgia's multi-symptomatic nature into consideration.

• Researchers have proven the FIQ to be valid and reliable (that is, it is able to measure what it is supposed to measure).

### How to Use the FIQ

As a fibromyalgia sufferer, you and your treatment team can use the FIQ to:

• Monitor your fibromyalgia progress.

• Document progress in measurable, quantifiable terms. This will also be crucial for your treatment to receive payment from insurance companies. These companies habitually deny claims for chronic pain cases.

Table 18-1: Fibromyalgia Impact Questionnaire

Name:_____

Date: _____

Instructions: For questions 1 through 10, please check the number that best describes how you did overall for the past week. If you don't normally do something that is asked, check N/A.

1.   WERE YOU ABLE TO:                              Always
Most Times Occasionally Never  Not Applicable

a. Do shopping?          ☐ 0   ☐ 1        ☐ 2       ☐ 3
☐ N/A

b. Do laundry with a washer and dryer?        ☐ 0    ☐ 1
☐ 2      ☐ 3      ☐ N/A

c. Prepare meals?        ☐ 0   ☐ 1        ☐ 2       ☐ 3
☐ N/A

d. Wash dishes/cooking utensils by hand? ☐ 0   ☐ 1
☐ 2      ☐ 3    ☐ N/A

e. Vacuum a rug?         ☐ 0   ☐ 1        ☐ 2       ☐ 3
☐ N/A

f. Make beds?  ☐ 0   ☐ 1        ☐ 2       ☐ 3       ☐ N/A

g. Walk several blocks?☐ 0   ☐ 1        ☐ 2       ☐ 3
☐ N/A

h. Visit friends and relatives?   ☐ 0   ☐ 1        ☐ 2
☐ 3       ☐ N/A

i. Do yard work?         ☐ 0   ☐ 1        ☐ 2       ☐ 3
☐ N/A

j. Drive a car?  ☐ 0   ☐ 1        ☐ 2       ☐ 3       ☐ N/A

2.   Of the days in the past week, how many days did you feel good?

☐ 0     ☐ 1     ☐ 2     ☐ 3     ☐ 4     ☐
5     ☐ 6    ☐ 7

3.   How many days last week did you miss work because of your fibromyalgia? If you don't have a job outside the home, check N/A.

☐ 0     ☐ 1     ☐ 2     ☐ 3     ☐ 4     ☐
5     ☐ N/A

Instructions: For the following items, place a mark like this ☐ at the point on the line that best indicates how you felt for the past week. You can also use numbers, like a scale of 1 to 10, 10 being the high end of the scale.

4.  When you did go to work, how much did pain or other symptoms of your fibromyalgia interfere with your ability to do your job?

| | | |
|---|---|---|
| No problem with work | --------------------------- | Great   difficult with work |

5.  How bad has your pain been?

| | | |
|---|---|---|
| No pain | --------------------------- | Very severe pain |

6.  How tired have you been?

| | |
|---|---|
| No tiredness | Very tired |

7.  How have you felt when you get up in the morning?

| | |
|---|---|
| Awoke     well rested | very tired |

8.  How bad has your stiffness been?

| | |
|---|---|
| No stiffness | Very stiff |

9.  How nervous or anxious have you felt?

| | |
|---|---|
| Not tense | Very tense |

10. How depressed or blue have you felt?

Not depressed                        Very depressed

11. Please indicate if you are taking any of the following for fibromyalgia:

☐ Tricyclics                        ☐ Anti-inflammatory
☐ Other central nervous system medications        ☐ Analgesic

☐ SAM e or any other nutritional product

Modified from: Journal of Rheumatology. (1991). 18, 728-733.

The Social Security Administration (SSA) and the Disability Insurance Program

## Table 18-2: Social Security Administration Criteria for Disability Determination

The claimant must be unable to "engage in any substantial gainful activity by reason of a medically determinable physical or medical impairment which can be expected to result in death or can be expected to last for a continuous period of at least 12 months."

The patient must have an impairment: "a demonstrable anatomy loss or abnormality of psychologic, physiologic or anatomic structures or function."

The impairment must be "demonstrable by medically acceptable clinical and laboratory diagnostic techniques. Symptoms alone cannot define an impairment."

From Social Security Regulations, 1986.

"Substantial gainful activity" is regarded as working on a job on a regular payroll of at least $700/month.

## Frequently Asked Questions and Answers About Disability Insurance

Q: What are "SSDI" and "SSI"? Are they similar?

A: "SSDI" is an abbreviation for "Social Security Disability Insurance," while "SSI" stands for "Supplemental Security Income."

The "SSDI" is a disability insurance program sponsored by the Social Security Administration (SSA) for workers who had worked for at least 5 years of the 10 years before becoming disabled. The program is funded by the "FICA" tax withheld from your paycheck.

The "SSI" is similar to "SSDI" and the SSA uses similar prequalification guidelines to administer both. The only difference is on the financial qualification requirement.

Furthermore, the benefits amount paid by the "SSDI" is influenced by your length of employment and salary level, whereas the "SSI" only pays a certain fixed amount before government-required deductions.

Some states may have other programs that can supplement the SSDI.

Q: Does 'other' or 'supplementary' income affect the amount of disability payments you receive?

A: According to Social Security and disability attorney Scott Davis, it shouldn't, since it is based solely on your income in your previous job. That is, investment income, for example, doesn't count. Also, your spouse's income will not affect your SSDI payments. However, it will affect your SSI benefits, since this is a welfare program.

Q: How are SSDI, state disability insurance, Workers Compensation and private insurance programs related?

According to attorney Scott Davis, the following states offer programs for illnesses and disabilities not caused by work: New Jersey, New York, Rhode Island, Hawaii, California and Puerto Rico. These states provide assistance before the SSDI program kicks in. Amounts paid are usually small and limited in duration, like 26 weeks in New Jersey and Hawaii. Please call your state's appropriate agency for further details.

Workers Compensation programs require that your illness be work-related, which the SSDI doesn't require. However, the SSDI requires you to have been unable to work for at least 12 months. Workers Compensation can pay for partial disability, but the SSDI requires you to be totally disabled before you can become eligible.

Private Disability Insurance: This is often provided by your company or you can fund it privately. Payment arrangements depend on the agreement in your policy. They may start disbursing benefits before any government programs. Amounts paid by private disability insurance may or may not be affected by the SSA benefits you receive.

Q: How do I know which type to apply for?

A: The Social Security Administration automatically determines which program you are qualified for.

Q: Can I continue to receive SSDI benefits after I attain the retirement age of 65?

A: The SSDI benefits cease when you get to 65 years. At this time, your retirement and Medicare payments would take over.

Q: What happens if I have been self-employed? Will I be eligible for any benefits?

A: Yes, if you have paid your FICA and self-employment taxes. It is common for many self-employed persons to neglect to do this.

Q: How large can these government benefits get?

A: As large as $240,000 by age 65, if you started receiving $1,000 monthly benefits at age 45 (according to attorney Scott Davis).

**Application Package Requirements**

According to another legal expert on this issue, Mr. Potter, in order to ensure a successful outcome to the application process, all concerned parties (claimant, her physician and attorney) must work as a team.

There should be a tenacity of purpose – that is, you must be prepared to go all the way. According to him, the system seems set up to poke holes in your application. Therefore, complete and detailed documentation of relevant information is crucial. In other words, your application package must contain the following information:

- Medical diagnosis
- Past medical history
- Types of medications taken or being taken
- Present functional status
- The history, nature and severity of pain
- Past work history and current work capacity
- Family status and current financial situation
- Housing arrangement
- Recreational lifestyle before and after fibromyalgia
- How have you been coping with the problem

The SSA focused medical review is aimed at finding out if there is about 90% reduction in your ability to perform at a job. For you to be eligible for benefit payments, there should be sufficient evidence that your illness is chronic in nature.

Your documentation should also include poor concentration at work, memory impairments, chronic disabling fatigue, etc. It will be in the best interest that your doctor is aware of all the documentation needed right from the start.

### Ineligibility Criteria

You will be considered ineligible for the disability insurance program under the following situations:

1. You remain employed, even partially, in spite of fibromyalgia.

2. You were able to recover within 12 months of being diagnosed with fibromyalgia.

3. You have no definite medical diagnosis.

When is the Best Time to File?

If it looks like you won't be able to return to your job in 12 months, then file by the sixth month. The process is usually long and drawn out.

### Disability Claim Application Process

STEP 1: Initial Application

If you worked before and paid taxes, apply under Title II. If not, apply under Title XVI. Forward application at your local Social Security district office either in person or by calling 800-772-1213.

Once your application is received and reviewed, the Social Security Administration would start gathering needed evidence.

STEP 2: Request for Reconsideration

If the initial application is denied (expect this), file a request for reconsideration within 60 days. You must note the jurisdictional nature of the timing. It means they will throw out your application if you can't beat the 60-day dateline.

Send this application through your disability claims attorney at the Social Security Administration office. The SSA determines the maximum amount your lawyer can charge you for his services. Usually, attorneys get 25% of back benefits (from your illness onset) up to a maximum of $4,000. Miscellaneous charges (obtaining expert opinions, etc.) are not included.

STEP 3: Independent Examiner Evaluation

The SSA will then send you to be evaluated by their own experts, usually in contract with the SSA. You may be denied again based on the expert's findings. The SSA will then suggest other alternative employment.

STEP 4: Request for Hearing

After your request for reconsideration is denied, you will have 60 days (jurisdictional) to apply. Your case will then be forwarded to an Administrative Judge, who sets a trial date in about 4 months. That is, he sets a date after 4 months your case file has been on his table.

STEP 5: Trial

The trial is an evidentiary process where you are allowed to provide both written documentation and oral presentation. Your physician's notes are examined. If this judge also denies your application, having determined you are not disabled within the law's criteria, you will again be able to appeal his decision within 60 days.

STEP 6: Appeals

Your case goes before the appeals council, which can give its verdict within 7 months. If you lose (that is, if affirms the trial judge's judgement), you will have the right to file suit.

STEP 7: Filing of Suit

You can file a suit after your appeal has been denied by the appeals council at the United States District Court. You must be represented by a properly licensed attorney; that is, licensed to practice at the US District Court. This Court may judge in your favor, and reverse the Administrative Judge's ruling, or may return your case for a new hearing called a remand. This process involves an examination of all the evidence submitted with the initial application at the district office.

## Making Sure You Will Succeed

A very good way to make sure you will succeed is to make sure your physician writes detailed and complete notes. Your disability attorney will coordinate the efforts of all concerned in writing an appropriate narrative report.

Recently, there hasn't been good news about successful applications and claims payment awards. A recent news release by the offices of Seattle-based Steven Krafchick, Esq., on November

30, 1999, announced a court victory on behalf of a disabled woman.

This woman's disability payments had been cut off by her insurance company – Paul Revere. The woman, a 52-year-old former executive secretary, was diagnosed with fibromyalgia and chronic fatigue. Her policy promised her benefits if she became disabled up to 65 years of age.

However, if she is diagnosed also with "psychiatric disorders," benefits would then be limited to only two years. So after some time of receiving payment, her insurance, Paul Revere, sent her to their own experts, who promptly, like almost on cue, labeled her a "psychiatric case."

The judge, Robert Lasnik of the Federal Court in Seattle, gave judgement in her favor. According to the judge, the so-called expert, a neuro-psychologist, was not an MD, and did not consult the patient's physician. Neither did he review her complete medical history.

And so, this expert could not have been able to determine her functional and psychological status or her work capacity. Paul Revere was then ordered to reinstate her benefits and pay her all accrued back benefits.

# Chapter 19: Summary, Conclusions And Frequently Asked Questions

### Summary

I hope I have tried enough in separating facts from hype about SAM e and its role in the relief of fibromyalgia symptoms.

The theme of this book has been that fibromyalgia syndrome is a multisymptomatic problem that requires an equally multifaceted treatment approach, and SAM e and the self-care non-drug strategies amply fit into this treatment model.

It is my contention that in most cases, addictive medications for a chronic and poorly understood health problem like fibromyalgia create more problems than they solve.

Furthermore, that there is no fix-all single remedy for fibromyalgia; rather, an effective medical treatment model must include necessary lifestyle changes by the patient, patient empowerment self-care strategies and a multidisciplinary cooperation.

A recap of the important issues discussed would include:
• Pain can be helpful in prodding us to finally make health-enhancing lifestyle changes we may have been putting off.

• Fibromyalgia is characterized by and differentiated from similar conditions by pain that is generalized in more than one extremity, and the presence of so-called tender points.

• About 80% of all fibromyalgia sufferers are mostly women between the ages of 25 and 55.

• There is no conclusive evidence about what causes fibromyalgia, and scientists are not certain that it is hereditary. Children can also suffer from a type called juvenile fibromyalgia.

• Conventional pharmacological remedies are known to cause substantial side effects and withdrawal reactions and may cause more harm than good.

• SAM e offers a safe alternative that is as effective, but without the unpleasant side effects of conventional medications.

• Pain is a constant complaint of fibromyalgia patients who would like to exercise. But exercise is mandatory if you want to get better or improve your life quality. The book has offered a safe and effective exercise and fitness guide, that of course depends on your motivation, determination and perseverance.

• Nutrition is a very important aspect of fibromyalgia treatment. Many of the symptoms can be remedied by a well-planned diet and nutrition. The following supplements are particularly effective for fibromyalgia healing: folic acid, Vitamin B Complex, malic acid, magnesium, valerian root, NADH, CoEnzyme Q10, L-carnitine, ginko biloba, phosphatidyl choline, acetyl L-carnitine, feverfew, peppermint oil and psyllium.

## Conclusions

Can fibromyalgia be cured? The standard textbook response is a negative. But I think this is wrong. It is not useful for our patients. It removes hope. The truth of the matter is that we don't know enough of fibromyalgia, what causes it or how it progresses, to pass such a definitive judgement. More research studies are needed.

Also, there is still some controversy (especially between rheumatologists and neurologists) whether the term "fibromyalgia syndrome" is a true diagnostic term at all. But having a diagnosis that differentiates it from similar or more serious conditions can offer some reassurance to the patients.

Until a definite cure is found, SAM e offers a lot of hope to the six million Americans who suffer from fibromyalgia. SAM e, as we have shown, is involved in several metabolic processes that are fundamental to the body's natural self-healing systems.

## Some Frequently Asked Questions About SAM e and Fibromyalgia

Q: Can SAM e cure fibromyalgia?

A: SAM e alone cannot cure fibromyalgia. A multisymptomatic problem like FMS requires a multifaceted treatment method. SAM-e offers a safe alternative to conventional medications that are known to have unpleasant side effects and withdrawal reactions.

Q: How does SAM e relieve fibromyalgia symptoms?

A: SAM e may relieve fibromyalgia symptoms by indirectly influencing (through methylation and other metabolic processes) the factors that probably cause and maintain the condition of fibromyalgia.

Q: How can we supplement SAM e through dieting?

A: We don't actually supplement SAM e due to the following reasons:

1. "Active methionine" is very limited in living organisms. SAM e gets quickly used up once it gives away its methyl group.

2. SAM e is highly unstable, and easily breaks down when we store or process our foods.

Besides, too much ingestion of protein can cause the production of harmful metabolites like ammonia.

Rather, we can through proper dieting enhance the process of methylation. This can be achieved by eating a well-balanced diet of soybeans, seeds, lentils, eggs, and protein-rich foods like fish and meat products. You must also take adequate amounts of other supplements like Vitamin B12, B6, folic acid and TMG (trimethyl-glycine).

Q: When can somebody have low levels of methylation?

A: Methylation is known to decrease with the aging process and has been implicated as a possible causative agent in disease states like depression, Alzheimer's and Parkinson's.

Q: Do fibromyalgia sufferers have low methylation problems?

A: Yes, it is possible. Methylation has a kind of seesaw relationship with homocysteine formation and degredation. This means that an increase of homocysteine level in the body is a sure sign of low methylation level and vice versa. There is a recent scientific evidence that fibromyalgia patients may have high levels of homocysteine.

Q: Why are we only recently hearing about SAM e? Isn't it just another hype?

A: The main reason is that most of the clinical trials about SAM e were conducted in Europe, especially Italy. Unlike the United States, these countries are more open to alternative forms of treatment, which have always been practiced alongside conventional pharmacological remedies.

Q: Why is it advisable to take only the "enteric-coated" type of SAM e?

A: This is because SAM e is absorbed mainly through the intestine. Using an enteric-coated form allows it to pass intact through the digestive environment of the stomach.

Q: Why is it important to store SAM e properly in a cool and dry environment?

A: Because SAM e is highly unstable and is easily broken down by heat and moisture.

Q: How does SAM e actually work in the body?

A: SAM e's efficacy is due to its versatile chemical nature – that is, its ability to donate its methyl group to acceptor molecules, thereby forming beneficial compounds. These processes in which SAM e is involved include methylation, transsulfuration and many other lesser-known processes.

Q: How can SAM e relieve depressive moods of fibromyalgia patients?

A: By assisting through methylation in the production of several neurotransmitters which can affect mood-like transforming L-dopa into a mood-regulator called dopamine.

Q: How does SAM e relieve fatigue symptoms?

A: SAM e can boost energy levels by assisting in the production of creatine phosphate. Athletes are known to take supplemental forms of creatine phosphate as energy boosters during high-impact sports.

Q: Has it been clinically proven that SAM e can help fibromyalgia sufferers?

A: Yes, the following have been proven about SAM e and fibromyalgia in clinical trials:

1. SAM e was able to improve depressive moods and reduce tender points in fibromyalgia patients.

2. A six-week treatment of fibromyalgia using a daily dose of 800 mg was found to improve symptoms of fatigue, pain, morning stiffness and mood.

3. Another study also found that SAM e was more beneficial than TENS (transcutaneous electrical nerve stimulation) in treating pain and tender points.

Q: Since SMA e is so expensive, are there any other alternative supplements?

A: Yes, another methylation agent is TMG (trimethylglycine). The problem is that some scientists believe TMG may not be involved in the brain cell methylation process and so may not be an exact substitute.

Q: How does SAM e affect gene abnormality repair? This is regarded as a possible causative factor for fibromyalgia.

A: The probable explanation is that SAM-e, through methylation of DNA and RNA, activates or deactivates genes. Activated genes produce disease-fighting antibodies; deactivated genes regress tumors and cancerous growths. Besides, SAM e plays an important role in polyamine manufacture. These contain nitrogen that is needed in DNA synthesis and gene expression repairs.

Q: How can SAM e improve sleep quality for fibromyalgia patients?

A: Through methylation, SAM e reacts with serotonin to form melatonin. Secreted by the pineal gland, melatonin is responsible for synchronizing hormonal release, thereby regulating the so-called "circadian rhythm," in which daylight promotes melatonin release, while darkness suppresses is.

Q: Why is SAM e regarded as better and preferable to regular antidepressants?

A: SAM e has quicker action – as soon as 4 to 7 days.

SAM e leaves no side effects even at very high doses, and will not cause withdrawal reactions if you decide to stop taking it.

Besides, unlike antidepressants, it is not a foreign compound in your body, and may in fact promote beneficial metabolic processes.

## RESOURCES FOR HELP

Fibromyalgia Syndrome
Fibromyalgia Network
P.O. Box 31750
Tucson, AZ 85751-1750
(520) 290-5508 (telephone)
(520) 290-5550 (fax)

American College of Rheumatology

60 Executive Park South, Suite 150
Atlanta, GA 30329
(404) 633-3777

Arthritis Foundation
1330 West Peachtree Street
Atlanta, GA 30309
(404) 872-7100
(800) 283-7800

National Fibromyalgia Research Association Inc.
P.O. Box 500
Salem, OR 97308

Social Security Disability Advocates Inc.
23930 Michigan Avenue
Dearborn, MYI48124
(800) 628-2887

Social Security and Long Term Disability Insurance Attorney:
    Scott E. Davis (480) 367-1601
    Or harris.davis@azbar.org

Fibromyalgia Association of Central Texas
2505 Western Drive
Garland, TX 74042-5650
(972) 494-1253

Fibromyalgia Frontiers

Fibromyalgia Assoc. of Greater Washington
13203 Valley Drive
Woodbridge, VA 22191-1531
(703) 790-2324 (Phone)
(703) 494-4103 (fax)

Newsletters about Fibromyalgia
Fibromyalgia Network
Cost: $19
P.O. Box 31750
Tucson, AZ 85751-1750
(520) 290-5508
(800) 853-2929

Fibromyalgia Times
Cost: $25
P.O. Box 20408
Columbus, OH 43221-0990
(614) 457-4222

Fibromyalgia Wellness Letter
Cost: $24.95
P.O. Box 921907
Norcross, GA 30010-1907
(877) 775-0343

Resources for SAM-e
SAM-e can be purchased in most pharmacies, grocery stores
and several other retail outlets.

Life Extension Foundation
P.O. Box 229120
Hollywood, FL 33022-9120
(800) 841-5433

Nature Made
(800) 276-2878

SAM-e periodic on-line pricing and purchasing Websites (as of 12/6/99)

Source: www.immunesupport.com/compare.htm.

| Rank | Web Site | Price | Product |
|---|---|---|---|
| 1 | Immunesupport.com | $17.99 | SAM-e (20 Tablets) |
| 2 | Samsstore.com | $18.98 | SAM-e (20 Tablets) |
| 3 | Cordette.com | $18.99 | SAM-e (20 Tablets) |
| 4 | Drugstore.com | $18.99 | SAM-e (20 Tablets) |
| 5 | Mothernature.com | $18.99 | SAM-e (20 Tablets) |
| 6 | Southern Chester Count Pharmacy | $21.98 | SAM-e (20 Tablets) |
| 7 | LEF.org | $25.50 | SAM-e (20 Tablets) |
| 8 | Cwinstitute.com | $28.20 | SAM-e (20 Tablets) |
| 9 | Iherb.com | $30.00 | SAM-e (20 Tablets) |
| 10 | Lifesourcenat.com | $34.99 | SAM-e (20 Tablets) |
| 11 | Smart-drugs.com | $36.95 | SAM-e (20 Tablets) |

12  Vitanet.com     $37.50  SAM-e (20 Tablets)

13  Immunonutrition.com $37.77  SAM-e (20 Tablets)

14  Vitaminconnection.com $39.95          SAM-e  (20  Tab-lets)

## GLOSSARY

**Antioxidant**. A substance that prevents oxidation. An example is gluthation.

**Adenosine triphosphate (ATP).** The body's main energy molecule.

**Aminopropylation**. The process in which SAM-e donates a methyl group to produce spermidine and spermine. These substances are necessary for cell growth, differentiation, nerve tissue repair, etc.

**Antidepressant.** Any agent used in treating pathologic depressive states.

**Anti-inflammatory.** Any agent that reduces an inflammatory response and associated pain and swelling.

Atom. The smallest unit of an element. Atoms aggregate to form molecules.

**Acetylcholine (ACh).** The chemical transmitter of the nerve impulse across a synapse. It is also released from endings of parasympathetic nerves (cholinergic nerves) upon stimulation. Some of its actions include cardiac slowing, dilation of arteries, increased gastrointestinal activity.

**Autoimmune disease**. Any disease characterized by injury to the tissue caused by an apparent immunologic reaction of the host with his own tissues. This is different from autoimmune response, with which it may or may not be associated.

**Antianxiety drugs.** Drugs used to treat states of worry and anxiety.

**Autoantibody.** Antibody that is produced in and reacts with a person's own antigen.

**Akathesia (restless legs).** A condition that often occurs just before falling asleep. Usually occurs in people under stress, it is characterized by spontaneous, uncontrollable leg movements.

**Amino acid**. Organic acid containing one or more amino groups (NH2) and a carboxyl group (CO2H). These form the essential component of proteins.

**Alzheimer's disease**. A disease of the brain that is characterized by a progressive diminishing of cognitive functions, especially in areas of short-term memory.

**Biopsy.** The removal and examination of tissue from the living body for the purpose of diagnosis.

**CoEnzyme.** A nonprotein organic compound produced by living cells, which plays an important role in the activation of enzymes, eg, riboflavin.

**Cofactor**. A substance whose presence is required to bring about the action of an enzyme.

**Chronic fatigue syndrome.** A condition that is characterized by extreme and continuous fatigue.

**Controlled study.** A study in which one group of subjects is used as a basis of comparison with another group. The subjects are also called controls.

**Cortisol.** A steroid hormone isolated from the adrenal cortex. Provides resistance to stresses and maintains a number of enzyme systems. Also called hydrocortisone.

**Cysteine.** Amino acid that contains sulfur.

**Circadian rhythm**. Denoting the rhythm of biologic phenomena that cycle approximately 24 hours. Example: Cortisol secretion rises in early-morning hours, peaks by the time we awake, and falls in the evening.

**Catecholamine.** Amine compound derived from catechol, such as epinephrine and norepinephrine, which are involved with nervous transmission, vascular tone and other metabolic activities.

**Cirrhosis.** A liver disease which is irreversible. Liver tissues are damaged by agents such as alcohol, viruses and toxins.

**Demethylation**. Removal of a methyl group from any molecule such as DNA.

**Deoxyribonucleic acid (DNA).** The molecular basis of genetics. Responsible for gene expression.

**Delta sleep.** The deep phase of the sleep cycle. This is also known as the restorative phase of sleep, in which brain wave activity is described as "delta wave."

**Dopamine.** A neurotransmitter produced in the brain. Produced by methylation of L-dopa. Dopamine is a principal mood regulator.

**Double-blind study.** A study in which two types of interventions are compared, and neither the study participants nor the investigators know what the intervention is. The participants are not influenced by knowledge about the intervention.

**Deconditioning.** This usually occurs in people with sedentary lifestyles or who have been inactive and on bed rest for a long time. Some deconditioning effects include decreased cardiac output, vital capacity, work capacity, etc.

**Detoxification.** Removal of toxins from the body.

**DSHEA.** Also called Dietary Supplement Health and Education Act passed by Congress in 1994. This Act allows drug manufacturers to produce and market any supplement with a good safety record with an FDA prior authorization, as long as these companies do not make any outrageous claims about the efficacy of these supplements.

**Enzyme.** A protein molecule which is able to increase the rate of chemical reactions.

**Enteric-coated.** Tablets and capsules that are coated so they are not digested by the stomach environment and allowed to get to the intestinal tract.

**Free radical.** An atom or molecule with an unpaired electron that can trigger off a series of oxidative reactions. They can damage beneficial systems like proteins, fats, membranes, cells, etc.

**Fibromyalgia.** A chronic disorder characterized by persistent and widespread muscle soreness, stiffness, chronic fatigue and many other symptoms, markedly including well-defined painful spots called "tender points."

**Fibro-fog.** A memory and concentration impairment of fibromyalgia patients.

**Fibromyalgia Impact Questionnaire**. A self-administered functional outcome test for fibromyalgia patients in areas of depression, functional and work capacity, anxiety, sleep, pain, stiffness, fatigue and general well-being.

**Fibrositis.** A former name for fibromyalgia, it is the inflammation of fibrous or connective tissue of the muscles. As we now know, there is no inflammatory process in fibromyalgia.

**Glutathione.** Body's powerful antioxidant. It also detoxifies the liver. Glutathione seeks out toxins, attaches to them, thereby making them water soluble and able to be eliminated in the urine.

**Homocysteine.** A toxic amino acid that is a by-product of methionine metabolism.

**Histamine.** An amine that can cause bronchiolar constriction, arteriolar dilatation, increased gastric secretion and a fall in blood pressure.

**Irritable bowel syndrome.** A chronic condition which is characterized by abdominal pain, stomach upset, constipation or diarrhea.

**Integrative medicine.** A health care practice that addresses all of human problems in all of the physical, psychological and spiritual ramifications. It uses all available treatment techniques, which it integrates to treat the human person.

**Inflammation.** A tissue reaction to irritation, infection or injury, characterized by localized heat, swelling, redness, and pain, and can result in some loss of function.

**Juvenile primary fibromyalgia.** Fibromyalgia that affects children and has no associated conditions.

**Lipids.** A chemical name for fats and oils.

**Lyme disease.** A disease caused by the Borrelia burgdorferi bacteria, transmitted by deer ticks. Symptoms begin as a large red spot on the thigh or buttocks, trunk or armpit and expands to about 6 inches in diameter. Other symptoms include fatigue, fever, headaches, muscle pain and joint pain.

**Lupus.** A disease that is characterized by joint pain, fatigue, muscle soreness and skin rashes. There is also joint swelling, organ disease like blood in the urine. Laboratory study would indicate elevated blood sedimentation rates, depressed white blood cell count and increased anti-DNA antibodies.

**Libido.** Emotional and instinctual energies and desires, usually referring to the sexual instinct.

**Metabolism.** Refers to all the biochemical processes in the body that sustain life. Examples include fat metabolism.

**Metabolic pathway.** A step-by-step order in which biochemical processes take place in the body.

**Methionine.** Essential amino acid that is the building block for SAM-e and homocysteine manufacture.

**Methyl group.** A reactive unit of organic chemical compound, containing one carbon and three hydrogen atoms. It changes the nature of whatever molecule it gets attached to. For example, when attached to a section of DNA, it prevents any damages to the genetic code.

**Methylation.** The process in which SAM-e loses its methyl group to another acceptor molecule.

**Melatonin.** A hormone that is produced in the pineal gland with the assistance of SAM-e. It is responsible for regulating the sleep-wake cycle.

**Methyl donor.** Any substance that has the ability to lose its methyl group to another substance.

**Muscle spasms**. Uncontrollable muscle activity.

**Metabolites.** Harmful by-products of metabolism, like lactic acid produced during muscle action.

**Migraine.** A recurrent, intense headache, usually localized on one side of the head and characterized by nausea, vomiting and visual disturbances.

**Myofascial pain syndrome.** A painful condition of skeletal muscles, characterized by one or several painful sites or trigger points located within muscles or tendons. When these sites are stimulated by palpation, they produce pain in the area of the patient's symptoms.

**Neurotransmitters.** Chemical substances often referred to as chemical messengers. They are released from nerve cells to activate receptor sites in other nerve cells, and thereby propagate nerve impulses. Example is dopamine and norepinephrine.

**NSAID.** This stands for non-steroidal anti-inflammatory drug. They are often prescribed to relieve pain by reducing inflammation.

**Oxidation**. A chemical process in which electrons from one reactant (reducing agent) are transferred to another (oxidizing agent).

**Osteoarthritis.** A degenerative joint disease characterized by degeneration of articular cartilage and hypertrophy of bone, accompanied by pain. Pain increases with activity and subsides with rest.

**Private disability insurance.** A nongovernmental and privately sponsored insurance program for work disability.

**Polymyalgia rheumatica**. A condition that is characterized by severe pain and stiffness in the neck and in the muscles of shoulders and hips. It can be accompanied by another condition called temporal (giant cell) arteritis.

**PTSD (Post-traumatic stress disorder).** This is an anxiety disorder caused by the experience of an overwhelming, traumatic event, which the person later experiences again repeatedly.

**Phosphocreatine.** A creatine phosphoric acid compound, a major source of energy in muscle contraction.

Palpitation. A rapid or forceful heartbeat, which the patient feels.

**Protein.** Complex nitrogenous substance of high molecular weight which contains fundamental structural units known as amino acids. Protein is present in the cells of all animals and plants, and are intimately involved in all phases of chemical and physical activity of the cell.

**Proteoglycan.** A complex of polysaccharide and protein, present in structural tissues of vertebrates like bone, and also in cell surfaces.

**Prozac (fluoxetine).** An SSRI drug; main function is to increase the levels of serotonin in the body. Used to treat depression.

**Rheumatoid arthritis.** An autoimmune condition charactarized by symmetrical inflammation of joints, usually hands and feet.

**Reynaud's phenomenon.** A condition in which the small blood vessels constrict, thereby decreasing blood flow to the extremities. The fingers turn very white on exposure to cold.

**Rapid eye movements (REM).** A sleep phase characterized by rapid eye movements, high brain electrical activity, somewhat like that of an awake state.

**Serotonin.** A central nervous system neurotransmitter. Can also be released by blood platelets following injury. Serotonin plays a role in mood regulation.

**SSRI (selective serotonin reuptake inhibitors**). A group of antidepressants that act by decreasing levels of serotonin in the brain. Example is Prozac.

**SSDI (Social Security Disability Insurance).** It is a disability insurance program sponsored by the Social Security Administration for those who had worked for at least 5 years before becoming disabled.

**SSA (Social Security Administration).** A government agency that administers government-sponsored welfare programs.

**SSI (Supplementary Security Income).** A government-sponsored disability insurance program for workers. Similar to "SSDI" in eligibility criteria, but different on the financial qualification requirement.

**Syndrome.** Denoting a complex condition, often with other associated conditions.

**Sjögren's Syndrome.** A condition characterized by a distinctive type of dry mouth and dry eyes. There may be oral and swallowing problems. It is an autoimmune condition associated with arthritis, muscle inflammation, thyroid and kidney problems.

Sleep spindles. A sleep phase in which brain activity diminishes to occasional spikes.

**Substance P**. A polypeptide found in the brain, especially the substantia nigra. It is a sensory transmitter that mediates pain perception.

**Somatomedin.** A peptide present in plasma, formed in the liver or kidney. It can stimulate synthesis of protein, RNA or DNA.

**Transmethylation.** A process in which there is a transfer of methyl groups between methyl donors and methyl acceptors.

**Transsulfuration**. A process in which homocysteine loses its sulfur to produce the amino acids cysteine, taurine or cystathionine.

**Tender points.** Well-defined painful spots on the body.

**TMJ (temporo-mandibular joint)**. Fibromyalgia patients sometimes complain of pain in the jaw region which can radiate to other parts of the face.

**Tension headache**. A type of headache characterized by pain around the head and neck regions.

**TMG (trimethylglycine).** Also known as "betaine." A methylated version of glycine. Another efficient methyl donor.

**Uncontrolled study.** A research study in which investigators and subjects are aware of the intervention being administered.

**Withdrawal symptoms.** The unpleasant effects of stopping the ingestion of an addictive chemical substance.

**Whiplash injury**. A neck injury caused by the sudden jerking of the head forward and backward.

# NOTES, RECOMMENDED READING AND WEBSITES

Overview of Fibromyalgia

Adam, N., & Sim, J. (1998). An overview of fibromyalgia syndrome: Mechanisms, differential diagnosis and treatment approaches. Physiotherapy, 7(8).

Bennett, R. M. (1999). Emerging concepts in the neurobiology of chronic pain: Evidence of abnormal sensory processing in fibromyalgia. Mayo Clinic Proceedings, 74, 385-398.

Bennett, R. M., Campbell, S., Burckhardt, C., Clark, S., O'Reilly, C., & Wiens, A. (1991). A multidisciplinary approach to fibromyalgia management. Journal of Musculoskeletal Medicine, 8(11), 21-32.

Bennett, R. M., Clark, S. R., Campbell, S. M., & Burkhart, C. S. (1992). Low levels of somatomedin-C in patients with the fibromyalgia syndrome: A possible link between deep sleep and muscle pain. Arthritis and Rheumatism, 35 113-116.

Cote, K. A., et al. (1997). Sleep, daytime symptoms, and cognitive performance in patients with fibromyalgia. Journal of Rheumatology, 24 (10), 2014-2023.

Dreher, T. (1999). Fibromyalgia Seminar. Larkspur, CA: Fibromyalgia Center of Marin.

Goodman, C. C., & Boissannault, G. W. (1998). Pathology: Implications for the physical therapist. Philadelphia: W.B. Saunders Company.

Hudson, J. I., & Pope, H. G. (1996). The relationship between fibromyalgia and major depressive disorder. Rheumatic Disease Clinics of North America, 22(2), 285-303.

Hulme, J. A. (1997). Fibromyalgia: A handbook for self care and treatment (2nd ed.). Missoula, MT: Phoenix Publishing Company.

Moldofsky, H. (1998). Sleep, wakefulness, neuroendocrine and immune function in fibromyalgia and chronic fatigue syndrome. Rheumatic Diseases Clinics of North America, 22(2), 219-243.

Russel, I. J. (1998). Fibromyalgia syndrome: Formulating a strategy for relief. The Journal of Musculoskeletal Medicine, 15(11), 4-21.

Shaver, J. L., et al. (1997). Sleep, psychological distress, and stress arousal in women with fibromyalgia. Research in Nursing and Health, 20(3), 247-257.

Wolfe, H., Smythe, H. A., Yunus, M. B., et al. (1990). The American College of Rheumatology 1990 criteria for the classification of fibromyalgia: Repot of the Multicenter Criteria Committee. Arthritis and Rheumatism, 33, 160-172.

Yunus, M., Masi, A. T., Calabro, J. J., Miller, K. A., & Feigenbaum, S. L. (1981). Primary fibromyalgia (fibrositis): Clinical study of 50 patients with matched controls. Seminars in Arthritis and Rheumatism, 11, 151-171.

SAM e and Fibromyalgia

Baldessarini, R. J. (1975). Biological transmethylation involving S-adenosyl-methionine: Development of assay methods and implications for neuropsychiatry. International Journal of Neurobiology, 18, 41-67.

Baldessarini, R. J. (1987). Neuropharmacology of S-adenosyl-L-methionine. American Journal of Medicine, 83 (suppl. 5A), 95-103.

Berger, R., & Nowak, H. (1987). A new medical approach to the treatment of osteoarthritis: Report of an open phase IV study with ademetionine (gumbaral). American Journal of Medicine, 83(suppl. 5A), 84-88.

Cantoni, G. L. (1953). S-adenosylmethionine: A new intermediate formed enzymatically from L-methionine and adenosine-triphosphate. Journal of Biological Chemistry, 204, 403-416.

Chiang, P. K., Gordon, R. K., Tal, J., et al. (1996). S-adenosylmethionine and methylation. Federation of The American Society of Experimental Biology Journal, 10, 471-480.

Clouatre, D. (1999). All about SAM e. New York: Avery Publishing Group.

Cooney, C., & Lawren, B. (1999). Methyl Magic. Kansas City: Andrew McMeel Books.

DiBenedetto, P., Iona, L. G., & Zidarich, V. (1993). Clinical evaluation of S-adenosyl-O-methionine versus transcutaneous electrical nerve stimulation in primary fibromyalgia. Current Therapeutic Research, 53, 222-229.

Friedel, H. A., Goa, L. L., & Benfield, P. (1989). S-adenosyl-L-methionine. Drugs, 38, 3889-3917.

Gatto, C., et al. (1985). Analgesizing effect of a methyl donor (S-adenosyl methionine) in migraine: An open clinical trial. International Journal of Clinical Pharmacology Research, 5, 39-49.

Grassetto, M., & Varotto, A. (1995). Primary fibromyalgia is responsive to S-adenosyl-L-methionine. Current Therapeutic Research, 55, 797-806.

Grazi, S., & Costa, M. (1999). The European arthritis and depression breakthrough! SAM e. Rocklin, CA: Prima Health.

Guibidori, P., Galli-Kienle, J., Catto, E., & Stramentindi, G. (1984). Transmethylation, transsulfuration and aminopropylation reacions of S-adenosyl-L-methionine in vivo. Journal of Biological Chemistry, 259, 4205-4211.

Jacobsen, S., Danneskiold-Samsoe, B., Anderson, R. B. (1991). Oral S-adenosylmethionine in primary fibromyalgia: Double blind clinical evaluation. Scandinavian Journal of Rheumatology, 20(4), 294-302.

Mitchell, D. (1999). The SAM e solution. New York: Warner Books Inc.

Murray, M., & Pizzorno, J. (1998). Encyclopedia of natural medicine (2nd ed.). Rocklin, CA: Prima Health.

Osman, E., et al. (1993). Review article: S-adenosyl-L-methionine – a new therapeutic agent in liver disease? Alimentary Pharmacology and Therapeutics, 1, 21-28.

Salvatore, F., Borek, E., Zappia, V., et al. (1977). The biochemistry of adenosyl-methionine. New York: Columbia University Press.

Stramentinoli, G. (1987). Pharmacological aspects of S-adenosylmethionine: Pharmacokinetics and pharmacodynamics. American Journal of Medicine, 83(suppl. 5A), 35-42.

Tavoni, A., Vitalie, C., Benbardier, S., & Pasero, G. (1987). Evaluation of S-adenosylmethionine in primary fibromyalgia: A double-blind crossover study. American Journal of Medicine, 88(5A), 107-110.

Volkman, H., Norregaard, J., Jacobson, S., et al. (1997). D-blind, placebo-controlled crossover study of intravenous S-ade-nosyl-L-methionine in patients with fibromyalgia. Scandinavian Journal of Rheumatology, 26(3), 206-211.

Fibromyalgia Medications and Their Problems: How to Come Off Them

Breggin, P. R. & Cohen, D. (1999). Your drug may be your problem. Reading, MA: Perseus Books.

Garner, E. M., Kelly, M. W., Thompson, D. F. (1993). Tricyclic antidepressant withdrawal syndrome. Annals of Pharmacotherapy, 27, 1068-1072.

Johnson, J. A. & Bootman, J. L. (1995). Drug-related morbidity and mortality: A cost-of-illness model. Archives of Internal Medicine, 155, 1949-1956.

Lazarou, J., Pomeranz, B. H. & Corey, P. N. (1998). Incidence of adverse drug reactions in hospitalized patients: A meta-analysis of prospective studies. Journal of the American Medical Association, 279, 1200-1205.

Manasse, H. R. Jr. (1989). Medication use in an imperfect world: Drug misadventuring as an issue of public policy. Part I. American Journal of Hospital Pharmacy, 46, 929-944.

Manasse, H. R. Jr. (1989). Medication use in an imperfect world: Drug misadventuring as an issue of public policy. Part II. American Journal of Hospital Pharmacy, 46, 1141-1152.

Maxmen, J. S. & Ward, N. G. (1995). Psychotropic drugs: Fast facts (2nd ed.). New York: W. W. Norton and Company.

The Merk manual of medical information (home ed.). (1997). Whitehouse Station, NJ: Merck & Co., Inc.

Mindell, E. L. & Hopkins, V. (1999). Prescription alternatives. Los Angeles: Keats Publishing.

The USP guide to medicines (1st ed.). (1996). New York: Avon Books.

Wolf, R. M. (1997). Anti-depressant withdrawal reactions. American Family Physician, 56, 455-462.


Other Drug-Free Fibromyalgia Relief and Self-Care Strategies

Abraham, G. (1992). Management of fibromyalgia: Rationale for the use of magnesium and malic acid. Journal of Nutritional Medicine, 3, 49-59.

Balch, J. F. & Balch, P. A. (1998). A to Z guide to supplements. New York: Avery Publishing Group.

Berkson, B. (1998). All about B vitamins. New York: Avery Publishing Group.

Butler, G. & Hope, T. (1945). Managing your mind. New York: Oxford University Press.

Kisner, C. & Colby, L. A. (1985). Therapeutic exercise: Foundations and techniques. Philadelphia: F. A. Davis Company.

Netzers, C. T. (1999). Big book of miracle cures. New York: Dell Publishing.

Passwater, R. A. (1998). All about antioxidants. New York: Avery Publishing Group.

US Dept. of Agriculture; US Dept. of Health and Human Services. (1995). Nutrition and your health: Dietary guidelines for Americans – E-text (4th ed.). Washington, DC: Author.

Woodham, A. & Peters, D. (1997). Encyclopedia of healing therapies. New York: DK Publishing Inc.

Fibromyalgia Disability Issues

Burchhart, C. S., Sharon, R. C. & Bennett, R. M. (1991). The fibromyalgia impact questionnaire: Development and validation. Journal of Rheumatology, 18, 728-733.

Cathney, M. A., Wolfe, F. & Klienkeksel, S. M. (1998). Functional ability and work status in patients with fibromyalgia. Arthritis Care, 1, 85-98.

Mason, J. H., Simms, R. W., Goldenberg, D. L., et al. (1989). The impact of fibromyalgia on work: A comparison to rheumatoid arthritis. Arthritis and Rheumatism, 32, R7.

Potter, W. J. (1992). Helping fibromyalgia patients obtain Social Security benefits. Journal of Musculoskeletal Medicine, 9(9), 65-74.

Silverman, S. L. & Mason, J. H. (1992). Measuring the functional impact of fibromyalgia. Journal of Musculoskeletal Medicine, 9(7), 15-24.

Social Security Administration. (1986). Social Security regulations: Rules for determining disability and blindness. Washington, DC: US Dept. of Health and Human Services. Social Security Administration. Office of Disability, SSA Publication No. 64-014.

## INDEX

*See also Borrelio burgdorferi.*

## M

## N

**T**

## About the Author

Dr. Joseph K. Egbebike, Ph.D.,PT is a Health & Life Coach, also a Physical Therapist with over 30 years of clinical experience treating thousands of pain sufferers. He earned his Ph.D in Pathokinesiology from New York University in 1992.

Sign up for his free newsletter and research updates at:
http://myfibromyalgiacure.com

Made in the USA
Middletown, DE
10 January 2021